Kama Sutra:

The Modern Guide to Exploring Sensual Secrets for Transforming Relationships and Exploring the Depths of the Kama Sutra

Lewis Finan

Table of Contents

Introduction:

Welcome to a journey of passion, connection, and sensual exploration. Within the pages of this book, you will embark on a captivating adventure into the world of the Kama Sutra, a timeless guide that transcends cultures and generations, offering a profound understanding of love, desire, and intimacy.

"The Kama Sutra: The Modern Guide to Exploring Sensual Secrets for Transforming Relationships and Exploring the Depths of the Kama Sutra" invites you to rediscover the ancient wisdom of the Kama Sutra, adapted to suit the complexities of modern relationships. It serves as a roadmap to enhance your sensual experiences, deepen your connection with your partner, and ignite the flame of passion that resides within.

Often misunderstood as merely a manual of sexual positions, the Kama Sutra is, in fact, a comprehensive guide to living a fulfilling and harmonious life. Originating from ancient India, this sacred text explores not only the physical aspects of lovemaking but also delves into the realms of emotional intimacy, communication, and the art of seduction. It provides a holistic approach to relationships, emphasizing the balance between sensuality, love, and spirituality.

In "The Modern Guide to Exploring Sensual Secrets for Transforming Relationships and Exploring the Depths of the Kama Sutra," we have curated a collection of insights, practices, and techniques that fuse the essence of the Kama Sutra with the realities of contemporary relationships. Whether you are seeking to reignite the spark in a long-term partnership or looking to navigate the exhilarating landscape of a new connection, this book will serve as your trusted companion.

Through the pages ahead, you will find guidance on understanding and embracing your own desires, unlocking your sensual potential, and creating an atmosphere of trust and intimacy with your partner. We will explore the art of seduction, the power of touch, the importance of communication, and the myriad ways in which pleasure can be experienced and shared.

As you delve deeper into the depths of the Kama Sutra, you will discover that its true essence lies not only in physical techniques but also in the mindset and attitudes that underpin the art of lovemaking. This book will encourage you to adopt a more mindful approach to sensuality, inviting you to savor each moment and appreciate the beauty of the connection you share with your partner.

Embrace the transformative power of the Kama Sutra and embark on a voyage of self-discovery and profound connection. May this guide inspire you to explore new realms of pleasure, deepen your love, and create lasting and meaningful relationships.

Chapter 1: Understanding the Kama Sutra

In this opening chapter, we embark on a journey of understanding the Kama Sutra, exploring its origins, purpose, and the timeless wisdom it offers. We will delve into the cultural context in which it emerged, dispel common misconceptions, and lay the foundation for a deeper exploration of this ancient text.

1.   The Origins of the Kama Sutra

The Kama Sutra, believed to have been written by the sage Vatsyayana around the 2nd century CE in ancient India, is a profound treatise on the art of love and living. It draws inspiration from earlier works and oral traditions, synthesizing them into a comprehensive guide for individuals seeking fulfillment in all aspects of life.

2.   Beyond Sexual Positions

Contrary to popular belief, the Kama Sutra extends far beyond a mere catalog of sexual positions. While it does contain a section dedicated to the physical aspect of lovemaking, its primary focus is on exploring the multidimensional nature of human relationships, encompassing love, desire, sensuality, and spirituality.

3.   Holistic Approach to Relationships

At its core, the Kama Sutra advocates for a holistic approach to relationships, emphasizing the integration of physical, emotional, and spiritual connections. It recognizes the interplay between these realms and offers guidance on harmonizing them to create profound and fulfilling partnerships.

4. Cultural Context of Ancient India

To truly appreciate the Kama Sutra, it is essential to understand the cultural context of ancient India. During this period, a vibrant and diverse society flourished, characterized by intricate social structures, religious practices, and philosophical frameworks that deeply influenced Vatsyayana's teachings.

5. The Three Aims of Life

The Kama Sutra is rooted in the concept of the "purusharthas," which outline the four aims of human life: Dharma (duty), Artha (material wealth), Kama (pleasure), and Moksha (liberation). Within this framework, Kama is celebrated as a legitimate and essential pursuit, as long as it is pursued ethically and with reverence.

6. The Five Sensory Pleasures

According to the Kama Sutra, the pursuit of pleasure is not limited to sexual gratification alone. It recognizes five sensory pleasures, known as the "pancha-tantra," which include sight, sound, smell, taste, and touch.

The text provides guidance on how to engage and enhance these senses, enriching the overall experience of pleasure.

7.   The Concept of Rasa

Another fundamental aspect of the Kama Sutra is the concept of "rasa," which refers to the aesthetic experience of emotions. It emphasizes the art of seduction, the importance of anticipation, and the creation of an atmosphere that heightens the pleasure derived from each encounter.

8.   Love and Communication

Communication is the lifeblood of any relationship, and the Kama Sutra recognizes its significance. It emphasizes the importance of understanding one's partner, fostering open and honest dialogue, and actively listening to their desires and needs.

9.   Gender Dynamics and Equality

While the Kama Sutra was written in a historical context with different societal norms, it does contain certain aspects that may be perceived as imbalanced in terms of gender dynamics. It is important to approach the text critically, recognizing the cultural context and extracting the valuable insights it offers while promoting equality and consent in modern relationships.

10. Ethical Considerations

Central to the teachings of the Kama Sutra is the notion of ethical conduct. The text emphasizes the importance of consent, respect, and consideration for one's partner, as well as the ethical responsibilities that come with exploring pleasure and desire.

In this introductory chapter, we have laid the groundwork for a deeper understanding of the Kama Sutra. We have explored its origins, clarified its purpose, and highlighted the multifaceted nature of this ancient text. As we move forward, we will delve into the practical applications of the Kama Sutra, examining the various aspects of sensuality, love, and intimacy that it encompasses. Let us now embark on a journey of exploration, embracing the transformative potential of the Kama Sutra to enhance our relationships and enrich our lives.

1.1 Introduction to the Kama Sutra

Welcome to the enchanting world of the Kama Sutra, a timeless guide to love, desire, and intimacy. The Kama Sutra is an ancient Indian text believed to have been written by the sage Vatsyayana around the 2nd century CE. It is renowned for its comprehensive exploration of human relationships and its profound understanding of the art of lovemaking. In this introduction, we will delve into the significance of the Kama Sutra, its historical context, and the enduring relevance it holds in modern times.

1. The Significance of the Kama Sutra

The Kama Sutra holds immense significance as a guide to a fulfilling and harmonious life. It goes beyond physical pleasure, offering insights into the depths of human connection, emotional intimacy, and spiritual transcendence. It explores the various facets of desire, love, and sensuality, aiming to create profound and transformative experiences within relationships.

2.   Historical and Cultural Context

To understand the Kama Sutra, we must explore its historical and cultural context. Ancient India was a land of rich cultural diversity, where philosophy, art, and spirituality thrived. It was within this vibrant setting that the Kama Sutra emerged, reflecting the social structures, religious beliefs, and philosophical ideologies prevalent at the time.

3.   Origins and Authorship

The exact origins of the Kama Sutra are shrouded in mystery, but it is widely attributed to the sage Vatsyayana. Vatsyayana drew inspiration from earlier texts and oral traditions, synthesizing them into a comprehensive treatise on love, desire, and relationships. Despite its ancient origins, the Kama Sutra's teachings continue to resonate with people across cultures and generations.

4.   Misconceptions and Stereotypes

The Kama Sutra has often been misunderstood and reduced to a mere manual of sexual positions. Such misconceptions overlook its profound teachings on emotional intimacy, communication, and the art of seduction. It is essential to move beyond stereotypes and explore the holistic wisdom that the Kama Sutra offers.

5. The Three Aims of Life

Central to the teachings of the Kama Sutra is the "purusharthas" or the four aims of human life. These aims include Dharma (duty), Artha (material wealth), Kama (pleasure), and Moksha (liberation). The Kama Sutra emphasizes the pursuit of pleasure within the ethical framework of one's duties and responsibilities.

6. The Multidimensional Nature of Love

Love, in the Kama Sutra, is a multifaceted concept that encompasses various dimensions. It explores romantic love, deep emotional connections, and the transcendence of self through love. The Kama Sutra encourages individuals to embrace love in all its forms and to cultivate relationships that nurture the soul.

7. Sexual Pleasure and Techniques

While the Kama Sutra is not solely focused on sexual techniques, it does dedicate a portion of its teachings to physical pleasure. It offers guidance on sexual positions, techniques, and the importance of understanding one's own desires and the desires of one's partner. The emphasis is on enhancing pleasure through communication, exploration, and creativity.

8.   The Importance of Communication and Trust

Open and honest communication is the cornerstone of any meaningful relationship, and the Kama Sutra recognizes its significance. It emphasizes the importance of understanding one's partner, expressing desires and boundaries, and actively listening to foster trust, intimacy, and mutual satisfaction.

9.   The Art of Seduction and Foreplay

The Kama Sutra celebrates the art of seduction and the role of foreplay in enhancing sensual experiences. It acknowledges the power of anticipation, the value of creating an ambiance, and the exploration of the senses to heighten pleasure and create a deeper connection.

10. Embracing Individuality and Diversity

The Kama Sutra recognizes that every individual is unique, with their own desires, preferences, and needs. It encourages the acceptance of one's own body and desires, as well as the celebration of the diversity that exists within relationships. It encourages individuals to explore their own sensuality and to honor the diverse expressions of pleasure.

As we embark on this exploration of the Kama Sutra, we are invited to embrace a holistic understanding of love, desire, and intimacy. The

Kama Sutra transcends time and cultural boundaries, offering profound insights into the human experience of connection and pleasure. Through its teachings, we can enrich our relationships, deepen our understanding of ourselves and our partners, and embark on a transformative journey of love and sensuality. Let us now embark on this enchanting path, guided by the wisdom of the Kama Sutra.

1.2 Historical Background and Origins of the Kama Sutra

To understand the origins and historical background of the Kama Sutra, we must delve into the rich cultural tapestry of ancient India. This chapter explores the socio-historical context in which the Kama Sutra emerged, the influences that shaped its development, and the profound impact it has had on human understanding of love, desire, and relationships.

1. **Ancient India: A Cultural Tapestry**

Ancient India, during the time when the Kama Sutra was written, was a land of diverse cultures, beliefs, and philosophies. It was marked by the rise and fall of empires, the flourishing of art, literature, and sciences, and a deep reverence for spirituality. This vibrant cultural tapestry provided the backdrop against which the Kama Sutra was born.

2. **The Vedic Period: Foundations of Indian Civilization**

The roots of Indian civilization can be traced back to the Vedic period, which dates as far back as 1500 BCE. The Vedic texts, composed in

Sanskrit, laid the foundations of Hinduism and provided insights into the social, religious, and philosophical values that shaped Indian society.

3.   Dharmashastras and Arthashastras: Codes of Conduct and Governance

During the centuries preceding the composition of the Kama Sutra, ancient India witnessed the development of texts known as the Dharmashastras (texts on ethics and moral conduct) and the Arthashastras (texts on governance and economics). These texts offered guidelines for personal conduct, social harmony, and the pursuit of worldly desires within an ethical framework.

4.   The Classical Period: Arts, Literature, and Philosophy

The classical period of ancient India, spanning from the 4th century BCE to the 6th century CE, witnessed a remarkable flowering of arts, literature, and philosophical thought. This period saw the emergence of influential schools of philosophy, such as Vedanta, Samkhya, and Yoga, which explored the nature of existence, consciousness, and liberation.

5.   Influences from Earlier Texts

The Kama Sutra drew inspiration from earlier texts and traditions, incorporating and expanding upon their teachings. It was built upon the foundations laid by earlier works, such as the Arthashastra of Kautilya

(Chanakya) and the Dharmashastra of Manu, integrating their wisdom into its holistic exploration of human relationships.

6.   The Role of Tantra

Tantra, a mystical and spiritual tradition that emerged in ancient India, had a significant influence on the development of the Kama Sutra. Tantra focused on harnessing and channeling energy, exploring the interplay between the divine and the worldly, and seeking transcendence through the integration of body, mind, and spirit.

7.   Vatsyayana: The Author of the Kama Sutra

The Kama Sutra is attributed to a sage named Vatsyayana, who lived in ancient India during the 2nd century CE. Not much is known about Vatsyayana's life, but his work, the Kama Sutra, has left an indelible mark on the understanding of human relationships and the exploration of sensual pleasure.

8.   Purpose and Scope of the Kama Sutra

The Kama Sutra was written as a comprehensive guide to the art of living, encompassing various aspects of human existence, with a particular focus on love, desire, and relationships. It aimed to provide individuals with insights and practical guidance for achieving fulfillment and harmony in their personal lives.

9. Manuscripts and Translations

The Kama Sutra was initially written in Sanskrit, and over the centuries, numerous manuscripts and translations have emerged. Some of these manuscripts were discovered in the 19th century, leading to a renewed interest in the text and its teachings. Translations into various languages have made the Kama Sutra accessible to a wider audience.

10. The Enduring Legacy

Despite being written over a thousand years ago, the Kama Sutra continues to captivate and inspire people in the modern world. Its teachings transcend time and cultural boundaries, offering profound insights into the complexities of human relationships, the exploration of pleasure, and the pursuit of a fulfilled and harmonious life.

The historical background and origins of the Kama Sutra provide us with a deeper appreciation of its wisdom and teachings. It emerged within the cultural tapestry of ancient India, drawing influences from earlier texts, philosophical traditions, and mystical practices. The genius of Vatsyayana, the author of the Kama Sutra, lies in his ability to synthesize these diverse influences into a comprehensive guide for living a life of love, desire, and fulfillment. As we continue our exploration, let us honor the historical context that birthed this remarkable text and embrace the timeless wisdom it offers.

1.3 Key Principles of the Kama Sutra

The Kama Sutra, an ancient Indian text attributed to the sage Vatsyayana, offers profound insights into the art of love, desire, and relationships. Beyond its popular reputation as a manual of sexual positions, the Kama Sutra encompasses a holistic approach to life, emphasizing the importance of emotional intimacy, communication, and spiritual connection. In this chapter, we will explore the key principles underlying the teachings of the Kama Sutra, revealing the wisdom it imparts for creating fulfilling and transformative relationships.

1. Understanding the Pursuit of Pleasure:

The Kama Sutra recognizes pleasure as a legitimate and essential pursuit in life. It celebrates the sensual and acknowledges that pleasure can be found in a multitude of experiences beyond sexual gratification. The text encourages individuals to explore and embrace the various dimensions of pleasure, whether through the senses, emotions, or intellectual stimulation.

2. Ethical Conduct and Respect:

Central to the teachings of the Kama Sutra is the principle of ethical conduct. It emphasizes the importance of treating one's partner with respect, kindness, and consideration. Consent and mutual agreement are emphasized, ensuring that the pursuit of pleasure is founded on respect for boundaries and the well-being of all parties involved.

3.   Embracing Individuality and Diversity:

The Kama Sutra recognizes and celebrates the unique desires, preferences, and needs of individuals. It encourages the acceptance and celebration of diverse expressions of love and desire. The text encourages individuals to explore their own sensuality, honor their desires, and create space for their partners to do the same, fostering an environment of acceptance and open-mindedness.

4.   Communication and Emotional Intimacy:

Clear and open communication forms the foundation of any successful relationship, and the Kama Sutra recognizes its significance. It emphasizes the importance of understanding one's partner, actively listening, and expressing desires, needs, and boundaries. Effective communication fosters emotional intimacy, deepens connection, and creates a safe space for vulnerability and growth within the relationship.

5.   The Art of Seduction and Foreplay:

The Kama Sutra celebrates the art of seduction and recognizes the importance of foreplay in enhancing sensual experiences. It encourages individuals to engage in playful and creative ways to arouse desire, prolong pleasure, and build anticipation. The text emphasizes the significance of creating an atmosphere that heightens the senses, allowing partners to explore and delight in each other's bodies and desires.

6. Mutual Pleasure and Satisfaction:

The Kama Sutra emphasizes the importance of mutual pleasure and satisfaction within intimate encounters. It encourages individuals to prioritize the pleasure and fulfillment of their partners, cultivating a sense of generosity and selflessness. The text highlights the reciprocity of pleasure, recognizing that by giving pleasure, one also receives pleasure in return.

7. The Role of Sensory Stimulation:

The Kama Sutra acknowledges the power of the senses in enhancing pleasure and deepening intimacy. It recognizes that sensory stimulation goes beyond touch alone and includes sight, sound, smell, taste, and texture. The text provides guidance on how to engage and enhance each of the senses, creating a more immersive and pleasurable experience for both partners.

8. The Importance of Forethought and Preparation:

The Kama Sutra stresses the significance of forethought and preparation in creating intimate and pleasurable encounters. It emphasizes the importance of setting the stage, creating an ambiance, and attending to details that contribute to the overall experience. This includes considerations such as grooming, personal hygiene, ambiance, and the thoughtful selection of appropriate settings for intimacy.

9.   Embracing Role-Playing and Fantasy:

The Kama Sutra recognizes the potential for role-playing and fantasy to add excitement and variety to intimate encounters. It encourages individuals to explore their desires, engage in imaginative scenarios, and indulge in consensual acts of role-playing that allow for the exploration of different roles, power dynamics, and fantasies.

10.   Continual Learning and Exploration:

The Kama Sutra encourages individuals to approach love, desire, and relationships with a mindset of curiosity, continual learning, and exploration. It emphasizes the ever-evolving nature of intimacy and the importance of adapting and experimenting to keep the spark alive in a long-term relationship. The text encourages individuals to seek new experiences, learn from each encounter, and nurture a sense of adventure and discovery within their relationships.

The key principles underlying the teachings of the Kama Sutra provide a guide for creating fulfilling and transformative relationships. By embracing pleasure, practicing ethical conduct, prioritizing communication, and exploring the senses, individuals can cultivate deep emotional connections and enrich their experiences of love and desire. The Kama Sutra invites us to embrace these principles and embark on a journey of continual learning, growth, and exploration in the realm of intimate relationships.

1.4 The Relevance of the Kama Sutra in Modern Relationships

The Kama Sutra, an ancient Indian text attributed to the sage Vatsyayana, may seem like a relic from the past, but its teachings on love, desire, and relationships remain surprisingly relevant in the modern world. Despite the vast changes in society and the evolution of cultural norms, the Kama Sutra offers timeless wisdom that can enhance and transform modern relationships. In this chapter, we will explore the relevance of the Kama Sutra in the context of contemporary relationships, highlighting its insights into communication, intimacy, self-discovery, and the pursuit of fulfilling partnerships.

1. Embracing Open Communication:

Effective communication lies at the heart of healthy relationships, and the Kama Sutra recognizes its enduring importance. In modern times, where communication can be hindered by distractions and technological barriers, the Kama Sutra emphasizes the need for open and honest dialogue between partners. It encourages individuals to express their desires, needs, and boundaries, fostering a deeper understanding and connection with their partners.

2. Nurturing Emotional Intimacy:

While physical intimacy often takes center stage, emotional intimacy is equally vital in modern relationships. The Kama Sutra emphasizes the significance of emotional connection, encouraging partners to cultivate trust, vulnerability, and empathy. In an era where the fast-paced nature of life can create emotional distance, the Kama Sutra reminds us to prioritize emotional intimacy as a foundation for long-lasting and fulfilling relationships.

3.   Exploring Sexual Expression:

The Kama Sutra's teachings on sexual expression continue to resonate in modern relationships. It encourages partners to explore and celebrate their sexual desires, fostering an environment of acceptance and open-mindedness. In a society that is becoming increasingly sex-positive and inclusive, the Kama Sutra reminds us to embrace the diverse expressions of sexuality and to communicate our needs and desires with respect and consent.

4.   Promoting Self-Discovery and Self-Awareness:

Modern relationships are greatly influenced by the quest for personal growth and self-discovery. The Kama Sutra recognizes the importance of self-awareness, inviting individuals to explore their own desires, boundaries, and preferences. It encourages self-discovery as a means to better understand one's own needs and to communicate them effectively within a partnership, leading to greater mutual satisfaction and fulfillment.

5.   Enhancing Sensory Pleasure:

In a world filled with distractions and constant stimulation, the Kama Sutra's emphasis on sensory pleasure is particularly relevant. It reminds us to slow down, be present, and engage our senses fully during intimate encounters. By prioritizing sensory pleasure, we can cultivate a deeper connection with ourselves and our partners, savoring each moment and enhancing the overall experience of intimacy.

6. Embracing Adventure and Variety:

Monotony and routine can dampen the spark in modern relationships. The Kama Sutra encourages us to embrace adventure and variety, providing inspiration for exploring new sexual positions, role-playing, and introducing novelty into the relationship. By stepping outside our comfort zones and embracing new experiences, we can keep the flame alive and maintain a sense of excitement and discovery within our partnerships.

7. Fostering Equality and Mutual Pleasure:

In an era of increasing awareness about gender equality and consent, the Kama Sutra's teachings on mutual pleasure and respect remain highly relevant. It emphasizes the importance of equal participation and prioritizes the pleasure and satisfaction of both partners. By fostering a sense of equality and shared responsibility, modern relationships can cultivate a more balanced and harmonious dynamic.

8. Embracing the Spiritual Connection:

The Kama Sutra recognizes the spiritual dimension of intimate relationships. It encourages partners to view lovemaking as a sacred act that transcends the physical realm, deepening the emotional and spiritual bond between them. In a time when spirituality and mindfulness practices are gaining popularity, the Kama Sutra reminds us to approach intimacy as a means of connecting with our higher selves and experiencing transcendence within the context of our relationships.

9. Honoring Individuality and Diversity:

Modern relationships are increasingly focused on celebrating individuality and embracing diversity. The Kama Sutra's teachings on accepting and honoring the unique desires, preferences, and needs of each partner align with this contemporary mindset. It reminds us to create a safe and inclusive space for partners to express their authentic selves, fostering a sense of acceptance, understanding, and celebration of diversity within relationships.

10. Navigating Modern Challenges:

The Kama Sutra's teachings offer guidance on navigating the challenges specific to modern relationships. It addresses issues such as the impact of technology on intimacy, the balancing act between personal and professional lives, and the need for self-care and self-love. By applying the principles of the Kama Sutra to these modern challenges, we can cultivate healthier and more fulfilling relationships in the face of societal changes.

The Kama Sutra continues to be relevant in modern relationships, offering valuable insights into communication, intimacy, self-discovery, and the pursuit of fulfilling partnerships. Its teachings provide a timeless guide for navigating the complexities of love, desire, and human connection. By embracing the principles of the Kama Sutra, we can enhance our relationships, cultivate deeper intimacy, and embark on a transformative journey of self-discovery and mutual fulfillment.

Chapter 2: Building Strong Foundations

Strong foundations are essential for building healthy, lasting relationships. Just as a solid structure requires a well-laid groundwork, successful relationships require a strong foundation to thrive. In this chapter, we will explore key elements and practices for building strong foundations in relationships. From trust and communication to shared values and emotional connection, we will delve into the building blocks that contribute to the longevity and fulfillment of partnerships.

1.   Trust as the Bedrock:

Trust forms the bedrock of any strong foundation in a relationship. It is the belief and confidence in one another's reliability, honesty, and integrity. Building trust involves being dependable, keeping promises, and being transparent in our actions and communication. Trust grows through consistent actions that demonstrate loyalty and respect, fostering a sense of security and emotional safety within the relationship.

2.   Effective Communication:

Open and effective communication is vital for building a strong foundation. It involves active listening, expressing thoughts and feelings honestly, and being receptive to your partner's perspective. Clear and respectful communication helps resolve conflicts, avoids misunderstandings, and strengthens emotional connection. It is important to create an environment where both partners feel comfortable expressing their needs, desires, and concerns without fear of judgment or rejection.

3.   Shared Values and Goals:

Shared values and goals create a sense of unity and purpose in a relationship. When partners align in their core beliefs, principles, and life aspirations, they build a foundation that supports growth and mutual understanding. Exploring and discussing values early on helps ensure compatibility and lays the groundwork for shared decision-making, compromise, and support in pursuing individual and joint goals.

4.   Emotional Connection and Intimacy:

Emotional connection and intimacy nourish the foundation of a strong relationship. It involves understanding and empathizing with your partner's emotions, being emotionally available, and creating space for vulnerability and deep connection. Emotional intimacy fosters a sense of belonging and strengthens the bond between partners, allowing for mutual support, comfort, and growth.

5.   Mutual Respect and Appreciation:

Mutual respect and appreciation are essential for building a strong foundation. Respect involves valuing your partner's opinions, boundaries, and autonomy, and treating them with kindness and consideration. Appreciation involves expressing gratitude for your partner's qualities, actions, and contributions. By fostering a climate of respect and appreciation, partners cultivate a positive and supportive atmosphere that nurtures the relationship.

6.   Conflict Resolution Skills:

Conflicts are inevitable in any relationship, but how they are resolved greatly impacts the foundation of a partnership. Developing effective conflict resolution skills involves active listening, seeking understanding, and finding compromises that honor both partners' needs. It requires a willingness to address issues openly and constructively, without resorting to blame or defensiveness. By resolving conflicts with respect and empathy, partners build trust and strengthen their bond.

7.   Quality Time and Shared Activities:

Spending quality time together and engaging in shared activities is crucial for building a strong foundation. It creates opportunities for bonding, creating cherished memories, and deepening the connection between partners. Quality time can involve engaging in hobbies, going on dates, or simply having meaningful conversations. By prioritizing time for each other, partners reinforce their commitment and create a sense of togetherness.

8.   Supportive and Equal Partnership:

A strong foundation is built on a supportive and equal partnership. It involves offering support, encouragement, and understanding to your partner's goals and dreams. A sense of equality ensures that both partners feel valued and empowered, with an equal say in decision-making and a fair distribution of responsibilities. Supporting each other's personal growth and ambitions fosters a sense of mutual growth and strengthens the foundation of the relationship.

9. Cultivating Individual and Collective Well-Being:

Building a strong foundation also requires nurturing individual and collective well-being. Each partner's self-care, physical and mental health, and personal growth contribute to the overall strength of the relationship. Taking care of oneself allows for a healthier, more fulfilling partnership. Additionally, investing in activities that promote shared well-being, such as exercise, mindfulness, or shared hobbies, strengthens the bond between partners.

10. Adaptability and Growth:

A strong foundation is built on the ability to adapt to change and embrace growth. Relationships evolve over time, and partners must be open to learning, adjusting, and evolving together. Building resilience and flexibility helps navigate challenges and transitions, ensuring the foundation remains strong even in the face of adversity.

Building a strong foundation in a relationship is essential for its long-term success and fulfillment. Trust, effective communication, shared values, emotional connection, and mutual respect form the core elements of this foundation. By nurturing these aspects and incorporating supportive partnership dynamics, couples can create a solid base that withstands challenges, promotes growth, and fosters a deep and lasting connection.

2.1 Establishing Emotional Connection

An emotional connection forms the essence of a deep and meaningful relationship. It is the bond that goes beyond physical attraction and shared interests, allowing partners to truly understand, support, and connect with each other on an emotional level. In this chapter, we will explore the importance of establishing emotional connections in relationships and discuss key practices and strategies to foster this essential aspect of intimacy.

1.   **Active Listening and Empathy:**

Active listening is a foundational skill for establishing an emotional connection. It involves giving your partner your full attention, being fully present at the moment, and genuinely seeking to understand their thoughts, feelings, and experiences. Through active listening, you demonstrate empathy and validate your partner's emotions, fostering a sense of trust and emotional safety. It is crucial to set aside distractions, practice non-judgment, and provide a supportive space for your partner to express themselves openly.

2.   **Expressing Vulnerability and Authenticity:**

Building emotional connection requires partners to feel comfortable expressing vulnerability and authenticity. Sharing fears, dreams, and insecurities allows for a deeper understanding and acceptance of each other's inner worlds. By creating an environment where vulnerability is welcomed and respected, partners can develop a stronger emotional bond and cultivate a sense of intimacy that goes beyond surface-level interactions.

3.   Emotional Availability and Responsiveness:

Being emotionally available and responsive is vital for establishing an emotional connection. It involves being attuned to your partner's emotional needs and providing support, comfort, and validation when they are experiencing difficult emotions or challenges. Emotional availability requires actively engaging with your partner's emotions, offering empathy, and being responsive to their emotional cues. By consistently showing up for each other emotionally, partners build trust and deepen their emotional connection.

4.   Sharing Life Stories and Experiences:

Sharing life stories and experiences is a powerful way to establish an emotional connection. By opening up about significant moments, personal history, and formative experiences, partners gain insight into each other's values, beliefs, and perspectives. This sharing of personal narratives creates a sense of intimacy, fostering a deeper understanding of each other's life journeys and fostering a sense of emotional connection based on shared experiences.

5. Cultivating Trust and Emotional Safety:

Trust is a foundational element of emotional connection. To establish trust, partners must create a safe and supportive space where vulnerability is met with compassion and understanding. Honesty, reliability, and consistency in words and actions contribute to a sense of emotional safety within the relationship. Building trust requires integrity, respecting boundaries, and demonstrating loyalty, allowing partners to feel secure in expressing their true selves.

6. Nonverbal Communication and Body Language:

Nonverbal communication and body language play a significant role in establishing an emotional connection. Paying attention to your partner's nonverbal cues, such as facial expressions, gestures, and tone of voice, can provide insight into their emotional state and deepen your understanding of their needs and desires. Nonverbal cues also allow for the expression of affection, support, and reassurance, enhancing emotional connection on a subconscious level.

7. Shared Rituals and Emotional Intimacy:

Creating shared rituals and moments of emotional intimacy strengthens the emotional connection between partners. Rituals can be simple, such as sharing meals together, engaging in regular date nights, or having daily check-ins to connect and share experiences. These rituals provide opportunities for partners to prioritize emotional connection and nurture their bond consistently.

8. Compassion and Emotional Support:

Compassion and emotional support are fundamental for establishing an emotional connection. Partners should offer understanding, empathy, and support when their significant other is going through challenging times. This includes providing a listening ear, offering words of encouragement, and being a source of comfort and solace. Compassion allows partners to feel seen, heard, and understood, fostering a deeper emotional bond.

9. Emotional Intelligence and Self-Awareness:

Developing emotional intelligence and self-awareness is essential for establishing emotional connections. Emotional intelligence involves recognizing and understanding one's own emotions as well as the emotions of others. Self-awareness allows individuals to communicate their needs, desires, and boundaries effectively, enabling partners to respond empathetically and build an emotional connection based on mutual understanding.

10. Nurturing Positive Interactions and Gratitude:

Positive interactions and expressions of gratitude nourish emotional connection. Partners should intentionally create opportunities for positive experiences, such as engaging in activities they both enjoy or engaging in acts of kindness and appreciation. Expressing gratitude for each other's qualities, efforts, and contributions strengthens the emotional bond and fosters a sense of appreciation and connection.

Establishing an emotional connection is a vital aspect of building a fulfilling and long-lasting relationship. Active listening, empathy, vulnerability, emotional availability, and trust contribute to the deepening of emotional connections between partners. By nurturing emotional connection through shared experiences, rituals, and emotional support, couples can cultivate a strong emotional bond that forms the foundation for a truly intimate and satisfying relationship.

2.2 Cultivating Trust and Communication

Trust and communication are essential pillars of a healthy and successful relationship. Trust forms the foundation upon which a strong connection can be built, while effective communication enables partners to understand and connect with each other on a deeper level. In this chapter, we will explore the significance of cultivating trust and communication in relationships and discuss key strategies and practices for strengthening these vital aspects of partnership.

1. Building Trust:

Trust is the bedrock of any successful relationship. Cultivating trust requires consistent effort and commitment from both partners. Here are some key strategies to build and nurture trust:

a. Honesty and Transparency: Honesty is crucial in fostering trust. Partners should strive to be open and transparent with each other, sharing their thoughts, feelings, and experiences honestly. Avoiding deception or hiding information helps establish an atmosphere of trust and authenticity.

b. Reliability and Consistency: Being reliable and consistent in words and actions is essential for building trust. When partners consistently follow through on their commitments, keep their promises, and show up for each other, it strengthens the belief that they can be relied upon and trusted.

c. Respect for Boundaries: Respecting each other's boundaries is vital for building trust. Partners should honor personal boundaries, both physical and emotional, and avoid crossing them without consent. Respecting boundaries fosters a sense of safety and shows that each partner's autonomy and comfort are valued.

d. Trust-Building Activities: Engaging in trust-building activities can strengthen the bond between partners. These activities can include exercises focused on vulnerability, such as sharing personal stories or engaging in trust exercises that require partners to rely on each other's support and cooperation.

e. Patience and Understanding: Trust takes time to develop and cannot be forced. Partners should practice patience and understanding, allowing trust to grow naturally over time. It is important to recognize that trust is built through consistent actions and behaviors rather than instantaneously.

2. Effective Communication:

Effective communication is crucial for understanding and connecting with your partner. Here are key strategies for cultivating effective communication in your relationship:

a. Active Listening: Active listening involves giving your partner your full attention, and focusing on understanding their words, emotions, and perspectives. It requires being fully present, avoiding distractions, and genuinely seeking to comprehend and empathize with what your partner is expressing.

b. Open and Honest Expression: Encouraging open and honest expression within the relationship is vital. Partners should create a safe and non-judgmental space where both individuals feel comfortable sharing their thoughts, feelings, and concerns without fear of criticism or rejection.

c. Non-Defensive and Non-Blaming Attitude: Effective communication requires adopting a non-defensive and non-blaming attitude. Partners should strive to approach discussions and conflicts with an open mind, seeking understanding rather than assigning blame. This promotes constructive dialogue and helps avoid escalating conflicts.

d. Clear and Assertive Communication: Clear and assertive communication involves expressing oneself in a direct and respectful manner. It is important to use "I" statements to express thoughts and feelings, focusing on expressing needs and desires rather than attacking or criticizing the other person.

e. Empathy and Validation: Practicing empathy and validation in communication builds emotional connection. Partners should strive to understand and validate each other's emotions, demonstrating empathy and support. This creates a sense of emotional safety and strengthens the bond between partners.

f. Conflict Resolution Skills: Conflict is inevitable in any relationship, and having effective conflict resolution skills is crucial. Partners should learn techniques such as active listening, compromise, and seeking win-win solutions. It is important to approach conflicts as opportunities for growth and understanding rather than as a means to win or control.

g. Regular Check-Ins and Quality Time: Regular check-ins and quality time dedicated to open and meaningful conversation foster effective communication. Partners should create opportunities to

discuss their relationship, share experiences, and address any concerns or issues that may arise.
h. Seek Professional Help if Needed: If communication challenges persist or become overwhelming, seeking the assistance of a relationship counselor or therapist can be beneficial. Professional guidance can provide tools and techniques to improve communication and resolve underlying issues.

3. Trust and Communication Feedback Loop:

Trust and communication are deeply intertwined. They rely on each other for growth and reinforcement. A strong feedback loop between trust and communication can be established by:

a. Trust as a Foundation: Trust provides the basis for open and honest communication. When partners feel safe and secure in their relationship, they are more likely to express themselves openly and authentically.
b. Communication as a Tool for Building Trust: Effective communication plays a significant role in building and maintaining trust. Open dialogue allows partners to address concerns, clarify misunderstandings, and establish a shared understanding.
c. Trust in Communication: Trusting that your partner will listen, respect your perspective, and respond with empathy strengthens the communication process. When partners have confidence in each other's intentions and actions, communication becomes more productive and meaningful.
d. Communicating Trust and Appreciation: Verbalizing trust and expressing appreciation for your partner's trustworthiness can reinforce the trust between you. Recognizing and acknowledging

instances where trust has been upheld builds a positive cycle of trust and communication.

Cultivating trust and communication is essential for a strong and thriving relationship. Building trust requires honesty, reliability, respect for boundaries and patience. Effective communication involves active listening, open expression, empathy, and constructive conflict resolution. By nurturing these aspects, partners can establish a solid foundation of trust and create a communication dynamic that fosters understanding, connection, and growth in their relationship.

2.3 Nurturing Intimacy and Vulnerability

Intimacy and vulnerability are at the core of deep and meaningful connections in relationships. Nurturing these aspects allows partners to truly understand, support, and connect with each other on a profound level. In this chapter, we will explore the importance of nurturing intimacy and vulnerability in relationships and discuss key practices and strategies for fostering these essential elements of closeness.

1. Understanding Intimacy:

Intimacy encompasses various dimensions, including emotional, physical, and intellectual intimacy. It involves a sense of closeness, trust, and connection between partners. Here are key strategies for nurturing intimacy:

a. Emotional Connection: Emotional intimacy involves sharing and understanding each other's emotions, thoughts, and experiences. Building emotional connection requires active listening, empathy, and creating a safe space for open and honest communication.

b. Physical Intimacy: Physical intimacy involves physical touch, closeness, and affection. Nurturing physical intimacy requires engaging in acts of affection, such as cuddling, holding hands, or engaging in intimate moments of physical connection.

c. Intellectual Connection: Intellectual intimacy involves stimulating conversations, sharing ideas, and engaging in activities that challenge and inspire each other's intellect. Nurturing intellectual connection involves actively seeking opportunities for intellectual stimulation, engaging in shared hobbies, and valuing each other's intellectual pursuits.

2. Creating a Safe and Non-Judgmental Space:

Creating a safe and non-judgmental space is essential for fostering vulnerability and deepening intimacy. Here are strategies to cultivate such an environment:

a. Trust and Emotional Safety: Trust is the foundation of vulnerability. Building trust involves consistency, reliability, and honoring commitments. Creating emotional safety requires being non-judgmental, providing support, and respecting each other's boundaries.

b. Active Listening and Empathy: Active listening and empathy create an environment where partners feel heard, understood, and validated. Practicing active listening involves giving full attention, avoiding distractions, and genuinely seeking to understand your partner's perspectives and emotions.

c. Non-Judgment and Acceptance: Being non-judgmental allows partners to express themselves authentically without fear of criticism or rejection. Accepting each other's thoughts, feelings, and experiences promotes vulnerability and encourages a deeper connection.

d. Compassion and Kindness: Cultivating compassion and kindness fosters an atmosphere of support and understanding. Partners should practice empathy, show kindness in their words and actions, and offer comfort and reassurance during moments of vulnerability.

3. Sharing Vulnerability:

Sharing vulnerability is a powerful way to deepen intimacy in a relationship. Here are strategies to encourage vulnerability:

a. Lead by Example: Leading by example and sharing your own vulnerabilities creates a safe space for your partner to open up. By demonstrating vulnerability, you show that it is acceptable and welcomed within the relationship.

b. Practice Active Listening and Validation: When your partner opens up and shares their vulnerabilities, practice active listening and provide validation. Validate their emotions, experiences, and perspectives to create a supportive environment where vulnerability is met with understanding and acceptance.

c. Avoid Judgment and Criticism: Judgment and criticism inhibit vulnerability. Avoid criticizing or dismissing your partner's vulnerabilities, as it can lead to them closing off. Instead, approach their vulnerabilities with empathy, understanding, and kindness.

d. Encourage Emotional Expression: Encourage your partner to express their emotions openly and honestly. Create opportunities for them to share their thoughts, feelings, and fears without fear of judgment or rejection. By fostering emotional expression, you create space for vulnerability and intimacy to flourish.

4. Cultivating Intimacy through Shared Experiences:

Shared experiences play a crucial role in nurturing intimacy in a relationship. Here are strategies to cultivate intimacy through shared experiences:

a. Quality Time: Dedicate regular quality time to connect and engage in activities that bring you closer together. This could involve going on dates, taking walks, cooking together, or participating in shared hobbies or interests.

b. Adventure and Novelty: Seek out new experiences and adventures together. Engaging in novel activities can create a sense of excitement and bonding as you navigate new territories together.

c. Create Rituals: Establish rituals that hold meaning and foster a sense of togetherness. This could include creating daily rituals like sharing meals or bedtime routines, as well as special rituals for anniversaries or celebrations.

d. Travel and Exploration: Traveling together allows for shared experiences, new perspectives, and opportunities to create lasting memories. Exploring new places can deepen your connection and provide a sense of adventure.

5. Emotional Support and Empathy:

Emotional support and empathy are vital for nurturing intimacy. Here are strategies to cultivate emotional support and empathy:

a. Be Attentive: Pay attention to your partner's emotional needs and cues. Be aware of their moods, stresses, and challenges, and provide support and comfort when they need it.

b. Offer Empathy: Empathy involves putting yourself in your partner's shoes and understanding their emotions and experiences. Show empathy by actively listening, validating their feelings, and offering comfort and understanding.

c. Communicate Love and Affection: Regularly express love and affection to your partner. Verbalize your appreciation, offer compliments, and engage in acts of kindness to show your care and support.

d. Be a Source of Strength: During challenging times, be a source of strength for your partner. Offer reassurance, encouragement, and a listening ear to help them navigate difficulties and provide a safe space to lean on.

Nurturing intimacy and vulnerability is crucial for fostering a deep and meaningful connection in a relationship. By creating a safe and non-judgmental space, practicing active listening and empathy, sharing vulnerabilities, and engaging in shared experiences, partners can cultivate intimacy and strengthen their bond. Building emotional support and empathy further enhance the connection, allowing partners to feel seen, understood, and accepted. Through the cultivation of intimacy and vulnerability, relationships can thrive and grow, creating a foundation for a fulfilling and lasting partnership.

2.4 Enhancing Emotional and Physical Compatibility

Emotional and physical compatibility are essential aspects of a fulfilling and harmonious relationship. Emotional compatibility involves shared values, communication styles, and emotional connection, while physical compatibility encompasses sexual intimacy and attraction. Nurturing and enhancing both aspects contribute to a deeper bond and overall relationship satisfaction. In this chapter, we will explore strategies for enhancing emotional and physical compatibility in a relationship.

1. Understanding Emotional Compatibility:

Emotional compatibility refers to the alignment of emotions, values, and communication styles between partners. Here are key strategies for enhancing emotional compatibility:

a. Shared Values and Goals: Shared values and goals provide a strong foundation for emotional compatibility. Discuss and align your beliefs, principles, and long-term aspirations to ensure that you are on the same page and working towards a common vision.

b. Effective Communication: Communication is crucial for emotional compatibility. Practice active listening, empathy, and open and honest expression. Create a safe space for both partners to share their thoughts, feelings, and concerns without judgment.

c. Emotional Connection: Nurture emotional connection by spending quality time together, engaging in meaningful conversations, and expressing affection and support. Regularly check in with each other's emotional well-being and offer support during challenging times.

d. Compatibility of Emotional Needs: Understand and meet each other's emotional needs. Recognize that individuals have different emotional requirements, and strive to fulfill them in a mutually satisfying manner.
e. Conflict Resolution Skills: Enhancing emotional compatibility involves developing effective conflict resolution skills. Learn to navigate disagreements respectfully, seek win-win solutions, and maintain open lines of communication.

2. Fostering Physical Compatibility:

Physical compatibility relates to sexual intimacy, attraction, and the overall physical connection between partners. Here are strategies for fostering physical compatibility:

a. Open and Honest Communication: Discuss sexual desires, preferences, and boundaries openly and honestly. Create a safe space for open dialogue about sexual needs, ensuring that both partners feel comfortable expressing themselves without judgment.
b. Exploration and Experimentation: Embrace a spirit of exploration and experimentation in the bedroom. Engage in open-minded discussions about fantasies, try new experiences, and remain receptive to each other's desires and interests.
c. Emotional Connection and Intimacy: Emotional and physical intimacy are interconnected. Cultivate emotional connection outside the bedroom to deepen physical compatibility. Strengthen the emotional bond through shared experiences, affection, and acts of love and appreciation.

d. Mutual Satisfaction: Prioritize mutual satisfaction in your sexual encounters. Focus on pleasure and intimacy for both partners, ensuring that each person's needs and desires are met and valued.

e. Continuous Learning: Sexual compatibility can evolve and change over time. Commit to ongoing learning and growth by staying curious and open to new experiences, as well as regularly checking in with each other's needs and desires.

3. Building Trust and Safety:

Building trust and safety is crucial for both emotional and physical compatibility. Here are strategies to establish trust and safety in your relationship:

a. Honesty and Transparency: Be honest and transparent with each other. Trust is built through consistent honesty and integrity in words and actions.

b. Respect for Boundaries: Respect each other's boundaries, both emotionally and physically. Communicate and establish clear boundaries, and honor them with understanding and respect.

c. Consent and Communication: Prioritize consent and open communication in all aspects of your relationship, including sexual encounters. Ensure that both partners feel comfortable voicing their desires and boundaries.

d. Emotional Safety: Create an emotionally safe environment where both partners feel secure expressing their vulnerabilities, fears, and insecurities. Offer support, empathy, and understanding when your partner opens up emotionally.

e. Reliability and Dependability: Be reliable and dependable in your actions and commitments. Consistency builds trust and creates a sense of safety within the relationship.

4. Nurturing Intimacy:

Intimacy goes beyond physical attraction and sexual compatibility. It involves deep emotional connection and vulnerability. Here are strategies to nurture intimacy:

a. Quality Time: Dedicate regular quality time to connect on an emotional level. Engage in activities that promote emotional closeness, such as deep conversations, shared hobbies, or simply enjoying each other's presence.
b. Affection and Non-Sexual Touch: Express affection through non-sexual touches, such as cuddling, holding hands, or hugging. These acts of physical closeness reinforce emotional connection and foster intimacy.
c. Expressing Appreciation and Gratitude: Regularly express appreciation and gratitude for your partner. Verbalize your love, acknowledge their efforts, and celebrate their positive qualities. This cultivates a sense of appreciation and fosters emotional intimacy.
d. Emotional Support: Offer emotional support and validation to your partner. Be there for them during challenging times, actively listen to their concerns, and provide comfort and reassurance.
e. Shared Vulnerability: Share your vulnerabilities and encourage your partner to do the same. Opening up emotionally deepens the level of trust and intimacy within the relationship.

Enhancing emotional and physical compatibility is a journey that requires continuous effort, open communication, and a genuine desire to strengthen the connection between partners. By nurturing emotional compatibility through shared values, effective communication, emotional connection, and conflict resolution, couples can deepen their emotional bond. Similarly, fostering physical compatibility involves open communication, exploration, emotional connection, mutual satisfaction, and building trust and safety. When emotional and physical compatibility is prioritized and nurtured, relationships can thrive, leading to increased satisfaction, intimacy, and overall relationship fulfillment.

Chapter 3: Sensual Exploration

Sensual exploration is an integral part of a fulfilling and passionate relationship. It involves embracing and celebrating the sensual aspects of intimacy, beyond the purely physical. In this chapter, we will delve into the art of sensual exploration, exploring strategies and practices that can enhance pleasure, deepen connection, and ignite a sense of adventure in your relationship.

1. Mindful Sensuality:

Mindful sensuality involves being fully present and engaged in the sensory experiences of intimacy. It allows partners to cultivate a deeper connection and heightened pleasure. Here are key strategies for practicing mindful sensuality:

a. Engage the Senses: Embrace all your senses during intimate moments. Pay attention to the feel of your partner's touch, the scent of their skin, the taste of their kisses, the sight of their arousal, and the sounds of their pleasure. Being fully present at the moment enhances the sensory experience.

b. Slow Down: Take your time and savor each moment. Slow down the pace of intimacy to allow yourselves to fully experience and enjoy the sensations. Let go of any distractions and focus on the present moment.

c. Non-Sexual Touch: Explore the power of non-sexual touch. Caress, stroke, and massage each other without the expectation of sexual activity. This type of touch fosters deep connection and relaxation, creating a foundation for more intimate experiences.

d. Sensual Exploration Activities: Engage in activities that awaken the senses and deepen sensuality. This could include activities such as blindfolded tasting sessions, sensual massages, or exploring different textures and fabrics together.

2. Erotic Communication:

Erotic communication involves expressing desires, fantasies, and boundaries with your partner. It enhances understanding, builds trust, and promotes a sense of adventure in the relationship. Here are strategies for cultivating erotic communication:

a. Create a Safe Space: Establish a safe and non-judgmental environment where both partners feel comfortable expressing their desires and fantasies. Encourage open and honest communication about sexual preferences and boundaries.
b. Share Fantasies: Share your sexual fantasies with each other. This can be an exciting and intimate experience that deepens trust and vulnerability. Discuss boundaries and explore ways to incorporate shared fantasies into your intimate experiences.
c. Use Sensual Language: Experiment with using sensual and erotic language to express your desires and fantasies. Verbalize what arouses you and what you find pleasurable. Communication plays a vital role in enhancing sexual chemistry and satisfaction.
d. Active Listening: Be attentive and actively listen to your partner's desires and boundaries. Show understanding, respect, and curiosity about their preferences. Validate their desires and offer reassurance that their needs and boundaries are valued.

3. Sensual Exploration and Playfulness:

Sensual exploration is an opportunity to embrace playfulness and creativity within your intimate experiences. It allows you to let go of inhibitions and discover new dimensions of pleasure. Here are strategies for incorporating playfulness into sensual exploration:

a. Try New Sensations: Experiment with different sensations to heighten pleasure. This could include using feathers, ice cubes, silk, or other sensory props. Discover what sensations ignite arousal and pleasure for you and your partner.
b. Role-Playing: Explore role-playing scenarios that excite and intrigue you both. Dress up, create characters, and embrace the opportunity to explore different dynamics and fantasies within a consensual and playful context.
c. Erotic Games and Toys: Incorporate erotic games or toys into your sensual exploration. There are various board games, card games, and sensual toys designed to enhance intimacy and ignite passion. Engaging in these activities can add excitement and novelty to your experiences.
d. Playful Teasing: Engage in playful teasing to create anticipation and build sexual tension. Teasing can involve light touches, whispered fantasies, or seductive gestures that leave your partner longing for more.

4. Emotional Connection and Sensuality:

Emotional connection is deeply intertwined with sensuality. Strengthening emotional bonds can heighten pleasure and intimacy in sensual exploration. Here are strategies to foster emotional connection in your sensual experiences:

a. Eye Contact and Intimacy: Maintain eye contact during intimate moments. Eye contact can deepen the connection and enhance the emotional intensity of the experience.

b. Expressing Love and Affection: Verbalize your love and affection during sensual exploration. Whisper words of adoration, express gratitude, and affirm your partner's beauty and desirability. This creates a sense of emotional closeness and enhances the sensual experience.

c. Emotional Check-Ins: Regularly check in with each other's emotional well-being during intimate moments. Ask your partner how they are feeling, what they enjoy, and if there are any boundaries or preferences they would like to communicate. This fosters open communication and ensures that both partners feel seen and understood.

d. Aftercare: Practice aftercare following intense or adventurous sensual experiences. Aftercare involves providing comfort, reassurance, and emotional support to your partner. It allows both partners to decompress, process their emotions, and reaffirm their connection after intimate moments.

Sensual exploration is an ongoing journey of discovery and connection. By embracing mindful sensuality, cultivating erotic communication, incorporating playfulness, and nurturing emotional connection, partners can elevate their intimate experiences to new heights. Remember that sensual exploration is a personal and consensual journey, and what works for one couple may not work for another. Embrace open communication, curiosity, and a sense of adventure as you embark on your own sensual exploration, deepening your connection and fostering a fulfilling and passionate relationship.

3.1 Expanding the Definition of Sensuality

Sensuality is often associated with the physical aspects of intimacy, but it encompasses so much more. It goes beyond sexual pleasure and embraces a holistic experience of pleasure, connection, and the celebration of the senses. In this chapter, we will explore the concept of expanding the definition of sensuality, incorporating various aspects of life and relationships that can contribute to a more fulfilling and vibrant experience.

1. Sensuality in Daily Life:

Sensuality can be experienced and celebrated in everyday moments. Here are ways to expand sensuality beyond the bedroom:

a. Mindful Eating: Approach eating as a sensual experience. Savor the flavors, textures, and aromas of your food. Engage all your senses while enjoying a meal, and appreciate the nourishment and pleasure it brings.

b. Appreciating Nature: Connect with nature and indulge in its sensual beauty. Take walks in parks, gardens, or natural landscapes. Observe the colors, scents, sounds, and textures of the environment around you.

c. Sensory Exploration: Engage in activities that stimulate your senses. Listen to music, dance, create art, or indulge in hobbies that bring you joy and evoke a sensory experience. Explore scents, textures, and colors that resonate with your senses.

d. Mindful Touch: Embrace touch as a way to connect and experience sensuality outside of sexual intimacy. Hug loved ones, cuddle with your partner, or enjoy a soothing massage. Focus on the physical sensations and the emotional connection that touch can bring.

2. Sensuality in Communication:

Communication plays a vital role in expanding sensuality in relationships. Here are ways to infuse sensuality into your communication:

a. Erotic Language: Incorporate sensual and erotic language into your conversations. Express your desires, fantasies, and admiration for your partner's physical and emotional attributes. Verbalize your appreciation and attraction to enhance the sensuality of your connection.
b. Flirting and Teasing: Engage in playful flirting and teasing with your partner. Use seductive words, gestures, or innuendos to create anticipation and build a sensual atmosphere. This type of communication can spark desire and enhance the connection between you.
c. Emotional Intimacy: Cultivate emotional intimacy through deep and meaningful conversations. Share your dreams, fears, and vulnerabilities with your partner. Emotional connection can heighten the sensuality of your relationship, creating a safe space for authentic expression.
d. Active Listening: Practice active listening to truly engage with your partner. Give them your undivided attention, show genuine interest, and respond with empathy and understanding. Listening attentively deepens connection and enhances the sensual bond.

3. Sensuality and Self-Care:

Self-care is an essential component of expanding sensuality. When we prioritize self-care, we nurture our well-being and create a foundation for a more sensual and fulfilling life. Here are ways to incorporate sensuality into self-care practices:

a. Sensory Bathing: Take luxurious baths or showers that engage your senses. Use scented bath products, indulge in soft towels, and light candles to create a soothing and sensual environment. Allow yourself to fully relax and enjoy the sensory experience.

b. Sensual Movement: Explore movement practices that awaken your senses and celebrate your body. This could include dance, yoga, tai chi, or any form of physical activity that allows you to connect with your body and its sensual capabilities.

c. Self-Exploration: Engage in self-exploration to better understand your own desires, preferences, and sensuality. This may involve self-pleasure, journaling, or engaging in activities that bring you joy and pleasure. By exploring your own sensuality, you become more attuned to your needs and desires within intimate connections.

d. Sensual Surroundings: Create a sensual environment in your living space. Choose fabrics, textures, and scents that evoke a sense of pleasure and relaxation. Surround yourself with beauty, art, and objects that resonate with your senses.

4. Sensuality in Non-Sexual Touch:

Physical touch is a powerful way to experience sensuality and deepen connections. It doesn't have to be explicitly sexual to be pleasurable and intimate. Here are ways to incorporate non-sexual touch into your relationship:

a. Cuddling and Embracing: Engage in cuddling and embracing without the expectation of sexual activity. This type of touch fosters emotional connection, intimacy, and a sense of security within the relationship.
b. Hand-holding and Massage: Hold hands with your partner and indulge in massages that promote relaxation and connection. Focus on the sensations of touch and the emotional bond it creates.
c. Sensual Exploration Activities: Engage in activities that prioritize non-sexual touch. This could include partner yoga, sensual massages, or simply exploring different textures and sensations together.
d. Non-Sexual Sensual Play: Playful touch and sensual exploration can exist outside of the sexual realm. Engage in activities such as tickling, feather play, or lightly tracing your fingers along your partner's skin. The focus is on the pleasure and connection that touch brings, rather than leading to sexual activity.

Expanding the definition of sensuality allows us to experience pleasure, connection, and fulfillment in various aspects of our lives. By embracing sensuality in daily life, infusing it into our communication, prioritizing self-care, and exploring non-sexual touch, we can create a more vibrant and fulfilling experience of sensuality. Sensuality goes beyond the physical, encompassing emotional intimacy, sensory exploration, and the celebration of pleasure in all its forms. Embrace the richness of sensuality and discover the depth it can bring to your relationships and overall well-being.

3.2 Awakening the Senses

The human experience is enriched through the senses. Our senses allow us to perceive and connect with the world around us in profound ways. Awakening the senses is a powerful practice that can deepen our appreciation for life, heighten our experiences, and cultivate a greater sense of presence and mindfulness. In this chapter, we will explore strategies and techniques for awakening the senses, allowing us to engage more fully with the world and enhance our overall well-being.

1. Sight:

The sense of sight allows us to perceive the beauty and intricacy of the visual world. Here are strategies for awakening the sense of sight:

a. Mindful Observation: Take time to truly observe your surroundings. Engage in nature walks, visit art galleries, or simply sit in a peaceful spot and appreciate the beauty around you. Notice the colors, shapes, and textures in your environment.
b. Engaging with Art: Explore various forms of visual art, such as paintings, sculptures, or photography. Allow yourself to be immersed in the art and let it evoke emotions and contemplation.
c. Color Therapy: Surround yourself with colors that evoke different moods and sensations. Experiment with incorporating vibrant and soothing colors into your living spaces, wardrobe, or daily accessories. Pay attention to how different colors make you feel.
d. Photography: Use photography as a tool to capture moments of beauty and curiosity. Take photographs of objects, people, or

scenes that catch your attention. This practice encourages you to pay attention to details and see the world through a different lens.

2. **Sound**:

Sound has the power to transport us, evoke emotions, and create deep connections. Awakening the sense of sound can enhance our experiences and bring us into the present moment. Here are strategies for awakening the sense of sound:

a. Mindful Listening: Practice active and mindful listening. Pay attention to the sounds around you, whether it's the chirping of birds, the rustling of leaves, or the melody of a favorite song. Allow the sounds to wash over you and fully immerse yourself in the auditory experience.
b. Music Appreciation: Explore different genres of music and actively listen to the melodies, rhythms, and lyrics. Experiment with creating playlists that evoke specific emotions or moods. Engage in music therapy practices such as singing, playing an instrument, or dancing to enhance your connection with sound.
c. Sound Baths: Participate in sound healing sessions or create your own sound baths. Use instruments such as singing bowls, gongs, or chimes to create soothing and resonating sounds that promote relaxation and mindfulness.
d. Nature Sounds: Immerse yourself in the natural sounds of the environment. Visit parks, forests, or bodies of water and listen to the rustling of leaves, the flow of water, or the songs of birds. Connecting with the sounds of nature can bring a sense of peace and grounding.

3. Taste:

Taste is a sensory experience that brings pleasure, nourishment, and connection. Awakening the sense of taste involves savoring flavors, exploring new culinary experiences, and embracing mindful eating. Here are strategies for awakening the sense of taste:

a. Mindful Eating: Slow down and fully engage with your meals. Pay attention to the flavors, textures, and aromas of the food. Take small bites, chew slowly, and savor each mouthful. Notice the subtle nuances of different ingredients and how they interact with your palate.
b. Exploring New Tastes: Step out of your culinary comfort zone and try new foods, spices, and flavors. Be open to experimenting with different cuisines and recipes. This expands your taste palate and introduces you to new sensory experiences.
c. Food Appreciation: Develop a deeper appreciation for the sources and preparation of your food. Visit local farmers' markets, grow your own herbs or vegetables, or participate in cooking classes to learn about the origins of the ingredients and the art of culinary preparation.
d. Mindful Tea or Coffee Rituals: Create rituals around tea or coffee consumption. Engage in the process of brewing, smelling the aromas, and savoring each sip. Allow the experience to be a moment of relaxation and sensory pleasure.

4. Touch:

The sense of touch connects us to the physical world and deepens our connections with others. Awakening the sense of touch involves engaging in tactile experiences that bring pleasure and connection. Here are strategies for awakening the sense of touch:

a. Texture Exploration: Engage in activities that allow you to explore different textures. Run your fingers through fabrics, touch various materials, or experiment with sensory objects like textured balls or fidget toys. Pay attention to the sensations and how they make you feel.

b. Sensual Massage: Incorporate sensual and nurturing touch into your relationships. Explore different types of massage, such as Swedish massage or aromatherapy massage, to create moments of relaxation and connection with your partner or yourself.

c. Nature Connection: Spend time connecting with nature through touch. Walk barefoot on grass or sand, feel the textures of tree bark or leaves, or immerse yourself in natural bodies of water. Let nature awaken your tactile senses and promote a sense of grounding and connection.

d. Self-Care Rituals: Engage in self-care rituals that involve touch. Take luxurious baths, use body oils or lotions, or engage in practices like dry brushing or exfoliation. These rituals not only nourish your skin but also promote a sense of self-love and well-being through tactile experiences.

Awakening the senses is a transformative practice that allows us to engage more fully with the world, heighten our experiences, and cultivate a greater sense of presence and mindfulness. By embracing the beauty of sight, the power of sound, the pleasure of taste, and the connection of touch, we can enrich our lives and deepen our connections with ourselves and others. Through mindful observation, active listening, mindful eating, and tactile exploration, we open ourselves to the wonders of the sensory world and discover new layers of richness and enjoyment in our daily lives. Embrace the awakening of your senses and embark on a journey of heightened perception and connection.

3.3 Pleasure Techniques and Erotic Arts

The exploration of pleasure and the erotic arts can deepen our connection with ourselves and our partners, expand our sensual experiences, and unlock new dimensions of pleasure and intimacy. In this chapter, we will delve into various pleasure techniques and the erotic arts, exploring practices that can enhance sexual pleasure, promote emotional connection, and ignite the spark of passion within intimate relationships.

1. Sensual Massage:

Sensual massage is a powerful technique that combines touch, relaxation, and sensuality. It can create a deep sense of intimacy, promote relaxation, and awaken the senses. Here are techniques to incorporate into sensual massage:

a. Setting the Mood: Create a serene and inviting atmosphere. Use soft lighting, scented candles, and soothing music to set the mood. Ensure the room is warm and comfortable to enhance relaxation.

b. Sensual Touch: Use a combination of techniques such as long strokes, circular motions, and gentle caresses. Vary the pressure and rhythm to create different sensations. Focus on areas like the back, shoulders, neck, and thighs, or explore full-body massage for a more comprehensive experience.

c. Incorporating Aromatherapy: Enhance the sensual experience with the use of essential oils. Lavender, ylang-ylang, and sandalwood are known for their relaxing and aphrodisiac properties. Dilute the oils in a carrier oil and use them for massage or diffuse them in the room.

d. Mindful Presence: Stay present and attuned to your partner's responses and needs. Check-in regularly to ensure their comfort and adjust the massage techniques accordingly. Encourage open communication to make the experience more pleasurable for both partners.

2. Tantra:

Tantra is an ancient practice that explores sexuality, spirituality, and connection. It emphasizes the integration of mind, body, and spirit to enhance sexual pleasure and deep intimacy. Here are some techniques derived from tantra:

a. Conscious Breathing: Deep, synchronized breathing can help cultivate relaxation and intensify pleasure. Practice conscious breathing together, synchronizing your breath with your partner's. This can create a profound sense of connection and enhance the energetic flow between you.

b. Eye Gazing: Engage in eye gazing to deepen intimacy and connection. Sit facing each other and maintain eye contact for an extended period. Allow yourselves to be fully present in the moment and observe the depth and beauty in each other's eyes.

c. Slow and Sensual Touch: Embrace a slow and mindful approach to touch. Explore your partner's body with curiosity and reverence. Focus on the sensations and the connection you share. By slowing down, you can heighten pleasure and build anticipation.

d. Energy Circulation: Explore techniques to circulate sexual energy throughout the body. This can involve visualizing the movement of energy or engaging in specific practices such as "microcosmic orbit" where energy is circulated between different energy centers in the body.

3. Role-Playing and Fantasy:

Role-playing and exploring fantasies can add excitement and novelty to intimate encounters. It allows for the exploration of different personas, power dynamics, and scenarios. Here are considerations for engaging in role-playing and fantasy:

a. Communication and Consent: Open communication is crucial when exploring role-playing and fantasies. Discuss boundaries, desires, and consent beforehand to ensure a safe and enjoyable experience for all involved.

b. Creating Characters: Develop characters and scenarios that resonate with both partners. Experiment with different roles, costumes, and props to enhance the immersive experience. Let your imagination run wild and embrace the opportunity for playful exploration.

c. Erotic Storytelling: Engage in erotic storytelling to heighten arousal and set the scene. Take turns narrating fantasies or creating a shared story together. This can build anticipation and create a sense of anticipation and connection.

d. Aftercare: After engaging in role-playing or exploring fantasies, ensure proper aftercare. Allow time for emotional debriefing, cuddling, and reassurance. This helps maintain a sense of emotional safety and connection after the intense experience.

4. Sensory Play:

Sensory play involves the deliberate stimulation of the senses to enhance pleasure and arousal. It can involve various elements such as temperature, textures, tastes, and smells. Here are some ideas for sensory play:

a. Blindfolding: Use a blindfold to heighten sensory awareness. By limiting sight, other senses become more acute, enhancing the pleasure of touch, taste, smell, and sound. Engage in sensual activities while blindfolded to intensify the experience.
b. Temperature Play: Experiment with temperature variations to stimulate the senses. Use warm or cold objects, ice cubes, or heated massage oils to create contrasting sensations on the skin. This can add an exciting element of surprise and arousal.
c. Food Play: Incorporate edible elements into intimate encounters. Explore the sensual pleasure of feeding each other fruits, chocolate, or other aphrodisiac foods. Experiment with taste combinations, textures, and temperatures to create a sensory feast.
d. Feather and Textured Fabrics: Explore the sensations of soft feathers or textured fabrics on the skin. Gently stroke, tease, or tickle your partner's body using these tactile elements. Pay attention to their reactions and adjust the intensity to maximize pleasure.

Exploring pleasure techniques and the erotic arts can enhance sexual experiences, deepen emotional connections, and bring a sense of adventure and excitement to intimate relationships. Whether through sensual massage, tantra, role-playing, or sensory play, these practices encourage exploration, open communication, and a deeper understanding of our desires and boundaries. It is essential to approach these activities with consent, respect, and a commitment to ongoing communication with your partner. By embracing the art of pleasure, we can create transformative experiences that enrich our relationships and ignite the fire of passion within us. Embrace the realm of pleasure and the erotic arts, and embark on a journey of self-discovery, intimacy, and pleasure.

3.4 Incorporating Tantra into Modern Relationships

Tantra, an ancient practice rooted in spirituality and sensuality, offers valuable teachings and techniques that can be incorporated into modern relationships. Tantra goes beyond conventional ideas of sexuality and focuses on deepening intimacy, cultivating connection, and expanding consciousness. In this chapter, we will explore how to incorporate Tantra into modern relationships, allowing couples to explore new levels of pleasure, emotional connection, and spiritual growth.

1. Cultivating Presence and Mindfulness:

Tantra emphasizes the importance of being fully present at the moment and cultivating mindfulness. In modern relationships, where distractions are abundant, practicing presence and mindfulness can significantly enhance connection and intimacy. Here are some techniques to incorporate into daily life:

a. Mindful Communication: Engage in mindful communication with your partner. Create a space where you can express yourselves authentically, listen actively, and respond with empathy. Practice deep listening, giving your undivided attention to your partner without judgment or interruption.

b. Conscious Touch: Embrace touch as a gateway to connection and presence. Engage in conscious touch by focusing on the sensations, and being fully present in the physical connection with your partner. This can be through gentle caresses, hugs, or simply holding hands.

c. Mindful Daily Activities: Infuse mindfulness into everyday activities. Whether it's cooking together, doing household chores, or going for a walk, bring your full attention to the present moment. Notice the sights, sounds, and smells, and allow yourselves to experience them fully.

d. Meditation and Breathwork: Incorporate meditation and breathwork into your daily routine. Set aside time to sit in meditation together or practice deep breathing exercises. This helps calm the mind, center yourselves, and cultivate a deeper sense of presence within your relationship.

2. Sacred Rituals:

Rituals create a sacred space and can be powerful tools for deepening connection and intimacy. Incorporating sacred rituals into your relationship allows you to honor the sacredness of your connection and create moments of intentional presence. Here are some ideas for sacred rituals:

a. Daily Gratitude Ritual: Begin or end each day by expressing gratitude for one another and your relationship. This can be done through spoken words, writing in a gratitude journal, or simply sharing a heartfelt moment of appreciation.

b. Couples' Meditation: Set aside dedicated time for couples' meditation. Sit facing each other, holding hands, or maintaining eye contact, and engage in a shared meditation practice. This allows you to synchronize your energies, deepen your connection, and cultivate a sense of oneness.

c. Tantric Bathing: Create a sensual and sacred bathing ritual together. Prepare a warm bath with aromatic oils, light candles, and play soft music. Take turns washing each other's bodies with love and reverence, allowing the experience to be a moment of deep connection and relaxation.

d. Sacred Space: Designate a specific area in your home as a sacred space. Decorate it with meaningful objects, crystals, and candles. This space can serve as a sanctuary for intimate moments, meditation, or connecting on a deeper level.

3. Exploring Energetic Connection:

Tantra recognizes the energetic aspects of our being and the potential for deep energetic connections between partners. By exploring and cultivating energetic connections, couples can tap into a profound source of intimacy and pleasure. Here are techniques to explore energetic connection:

a. Eye Gazing: Engage in eye-gazing exercises to deepen the energetic connection. Sit facing each other in a comfortable position and maintain eye contact for an extended period. Allow yourselves to drop into a state of deep connection and presence, sensing the energetic exchange between you.

b. Sharing Breath: Explore the practice of sharing breath with your partner. Sit or lie down facing each other, and synchronize your breath. Breathe in together, allowing your breath to merge, and exhale together. This practice helps synchronize your energies and create a heightened sense of connection.

c. Chakra Meditation: Engage in chakra meditation together. Visualize and focus on each of the seven chakras, starting from the base of the spine and moving up to the crown of the head. As you focus on each chakra, visualize it being balanced and energized, allowing the energy to flow freely between you and your partner.

d. Sensual Energy Exchange: During intimate moments, consciously exchange energy with your partner. As you engage in physical touch, visualize the energy flowing between you, connecting and merging your energetic fields. This can enhance the depth of connection and the intensity of pleasure.

4. Sacred Sexuality:

Tantra recognizes sexuality as a sacred and transformative aspect of human experience. It encourages a conscious and holistic approach to sexuality, going beyond the physical act and embracing the emotional, energetic, and spiritual dimensions. Here are some elements of sacred sexuality to explore:

a. Slow and Mindful Approach: Embrace a slow and mindful approach to sexual intimacy. Instead of rushing towards orgasm, focus on the journey and the connection with your partner. Engage in conscious touch, explore the sensations, and allow yourselves to fully experience the pleasure.

b. Extended Lovemaking: Extend the duration of lovemaking by embracing techniques such as tantric edging or non-goal-oriented lovemaking. This allows you to build sexual energy gradually and experience prolonged states of pleasure and deep connection.

c. Breathwork and Sound: Incorporate breathwork and sound into your sexual experiences. Use deep breathing to circulate sexual energy throughout your body, intensifying pleasure. Explore vocalization and expressing sounds of pleasure to deepen your connection and enhance the energetic exchange.

d. Transcendence and Connection: During sexual intimacy, aim for transcendence and connection beyond the physical realm. Cultivate an awareness of the energy flowing between you and your partner, allowing it to merge and expand. This can lead to profound states of bliss, connection, and spiritual union.

Incorporating Tantra into modern relationships can transform our approach to intimacy, pleasure, and connection. By embracing presence, sacred rituals, energetic exploration, and sacred sexuality, couples can deepen their emotional bond, expand their pleasure, and cultivate a profound sense of connection and spiritual growth. It is important to approach these practices with open-mindedness, consent, and ongoing communication with your partner. Through the integration of Tantra, couples can embark on a journey of self-discovery, transformation, and the exploration of new dimensions of love and intimacy. Embrace the wisdom of Tantra and allow it to enhance the richness and depth of your modern relationship.

Chapter 4: Deepening Intimacy and Connection

Intimacy and connection are the cornerstones of a fulfilling and thriving relationship. In this chapter, we will explore various techniques and practices to deepen intimacy and connection between partners. By nurturing emotional closeness, fostering vulnerability, and prioritizing deep connection, couples can cultivate a strong and enduring bond. Let us delve into the strategies and practices that can help couples create a deeper level of intimacy and connection in their relationship.

1. Emotional Vulnerability:

Emotional vulnerability forms the foundation of deep intimacy and connection. It involves being open, authentic, and transparent with our feelings, fears, and desires. Here are some ways to foster emotional vulnerability:

a. Safe and Non-judgmental Space: Create a safe and non-judgmental space for each other to express emotions. Practice active listening, empathy, and validation. Encourage open and honest communication, allowing each other to share thoughts and feelings without fear of criticism or judgment.

b. Sharing Personal Experiences: Share personal experiences and stories that reveal vulnerability. This can include childhood memories, past struggles, or moments of personal growth. By sharing our vulnerabilities, we invite our partner to do the same, deepening the emotional bond between us.

c. Expressing Appreciation and Gratitude: Regularly express appreciation and gratitude for one another. Acknowledge the qualities, actions, and efforts that you value in your partner. This fosters an environment of emotional support and validation, encouraging vulnerability and emotional connection.

d. Emotional Check-ins: Incorporate regular emotional check-ins into your routine. Set aside dedicated time to discuss emotions, concerns, and needs. This allows both partners to feel heard, understood, and supported, strengthening the emotional connection.

2. Deepening Communication:

Effective communication is vital for deepening intimacy and connection in a relationship. It involves not only expressing thoughts and feelings but also actively listening and understanding each other. Here are techniques to enhance communication:

a. Active Listening: Practice active listening by giving your full attention to your partner when they are speaking. Maintain eye contact, avoid interrupting, and show genuine interest in what they have to say. Reflect back on what you heard to ensure understanding.

b. Non-Verbal Communication: Pay attention to non-verbal cues such as body language and facial expressions. These can often communicate emotions that words may not express. Be mindful of your own non-verbal communication and strive to be open and receptive.

c. Empathetic Responses: Respond with empathy and understanding when your partner shares their thoughts or feelings. Try to put yourself in their shoes and validate their emotions. Avoid

becoming defensive or dismissive, and instead, strive to offer
support and comfort.

d. Conflict Resolution: Develop healthy conflict resolution skills.
Instead of resorting to blame or criticism, approach conflicts as
opportunities for growth and understanding. Use "I" statements to
express your feelings and needs, and work together to find
mutually beneficial solutions.

3. Cultivating Shared Experiences:

Shared experiences create a sense of togetherness and foster a deep
connection between partners. By intentionally creating and nurturing
shared experiences, couples can strengthen their emotional bond. Here
are some ideas to cultivate shared experiences:

a. Date Nights: Set aside dedicated time for regular date nights.
These can involve going out for dinner, taking a walk in nature,
attending events or shows, or simply enjoying a quiet evening at
home. The key is to prioritize quality time together and engage in
activities that you both enjoy.

b. Shared Hobbies and Interests: Discover and cultivate shared
hobbies and interests. Find activities that you both find enjoyable
and engage in them regularly. This could be cooking together,
practicing a sport, learning a musical instrument, or exploring a
new hobby as a team.

c. Travel and Adventure: Embark on adventures and travel together.
Explore new places, cultures, and experiences. Traveling allows
you to create lasting memories and strengthens the bond by
navigating new environments together.

d. Rituals and Traditions: Develop unique rituals and traditions that are special to your relationship. This could be a weekly movie night, a yearly getaway, or a meaningful celebration. Rituals and traditions create a sense of continuity and reinforce the shared history and connection.

4. Intimacy and Physical Connection:

Physical intimacy plays a crucial role in deepening connection and intimacy. It involves not only sexual intimacy but also non-sexual touch and affection. Here are ways to enhance physical connection:

a. Affectionate Touch: Engage in non-sexual touch throughout the day. Hold hands, cuddle, give hugs, or simply touch each other affectionately. Physical touch releases oxytocin, a hormone associated with bonding and intimacy.
b. Sensual Massage: Explore sensual massage as a way to connect and nurture each other. Set aside dedicated time for giving and receiving massages, using aromatic oils, and creating a soothing environment. This allows you to focus on each other's bodies and deepen the physical and emotional connection.
c. Intimate Conversations: Engage in intimate conversations about desires, fantasies, and preferences. Create a safe space where you can openly discuss your sexual needs and explore new avenues of pleasure together. This builds trust and understanding, enhancing the sexual connection.
d. Sexual Exploration: Continually explore and experiment with your sexual connection. Be open to trying new things, discussing fantasies, and engaging in activities that bring pleasure and

excitement to both partners. Open and honest communication about sexual desires can lead to increased intimacy and connection.

Deepening intimacy and connection is an ongoing process that requires intentional effort and commitment. By fostering emotional vulnerability, enhancing communication, cultivating shared experiences, and nurturing physical intimacy, couples can create a profound and enduring bond. It is important to remember that every relationship is unique, and the strategies that work best will vary. Explore these techniques with an open mind and adapt them to suit your specific needs and preferences. By prioritizing and investing in the depth of connection and intimacy, couples can create a relationship that is fulfilling, nurturing, and resilient.

4.1 Honoring Individual Desires and Boundaries

In any relationship, it is crucial to honor and respect the individual desires and boundaries of each partner. Recognizing and valuing each other's unique needs and boundaries is essential for maintaining a healthy and fulfilling connection. In this chapter, we will explore the importance of honoring individual desires and boundaries in a relationship, and provide strategies for effective communication, negotiation, and mutual understanding.

1. Understanding Individual Desires:

Every individual has unique desires, preferences, and needs. Honoring and acknowledging these desires is crucial for maintaining a sense of fulfillment and satisfaction within the relationship. Here are some key points to consider:

a. Self-Reflection: Encourage self-reflection and introspection in both partners. Take the time to understand your own desires, interests, and passions. This self-awareness will allow you to effectively communicate your needs to your partner.

b. Open Communication: Foster an environment of open and honest communication. Encourage each other to express desires, fantasies, and interests without fear of judgment or rejection. Actively listen and validate each other's desires, even if they differ from your own.

c. Sharing Fantasies and Dreams: Create a safe space for sharing fantasies and dreams. Engage in conversations about the things you both desire and explore ways to incorporate them into your relationship. This can be done through open dialogue, role-playing, or even creating a shared bucket list of experiences.

d. Continual Exploration: Recognize that desires and interests may evolve over time. Be open to exploring new experiences, activities, and interests together. Regularly check in with each other to ensure that desires are being met and adjust accordingly.

2. Setting and Respecting Boundaries:

Boundaries are essential for maintaining personal autonomy and emotional well-being. Each partner should feel comfortable expressing their boundaries and have them respected by their significant other. Here are some strategies for setting and respecting boundaries:

a. Self-Awareness: Encourage self-awareness regarding personal boundaries. Take the time to understand your own limits, needs, and comfort levels. This will allow you to communicate your boundaries effectively to your partner.

b. Open Dialogue: Foster open dialogue about boundaries within the relationship. Create a safe space for discussing what feels comfortable and what doesn't. Encourage active listening, empathy, and understanding when discussing boundaries.

c. Respect and Consent: Ensure that boundaries are respected at all times. Obtain explicit consent before engaging in any activity that may involve crossing personal boundaries. Consistently check in with each other to ensure that boundaries are being honored and adjust accordingly.

d. Flexibility and Compromise: Recognize that boundaries may vary between individuals and may require compromise. Engage in open conversations to find mutually beneficial solutions when boundaries differ. Strive for a balance that respects each partner's needs and ensures emotional well-being.

3. Effective Communication and Negotiation:

Effective communication and negotiation skills are essential for honoring individual desires and boundaries. Here are some strategies to facilitate open and respectful communication:

a. Active Listening: Practice active listening when discussing desires and boundaries. Give your full attention to your partner, maintain eye contact, and avoid interrupting. Show empathy and understanding by reflecting back on what you've heard.

b. Use "I" Statements: Use "I" statements when expressing desires and boundaries to avoid sounding accusatory or judgmental. Focus on expressing your own feelings and needs rather than criticizing or blaming your partner.

c. Seek Clarity and Understanding: Ask clarifying questions to ensure that you understand your partner's desires and boundaries fully. Seek to understand their perspective and validate their feelings. This promotes a sense of trust and mutual understanding.

d. Find Win-Win Solutions: Approach disagreements or differing desires with a mindset of finding win-win solutions. Strive for compromise and collaboration that respects both partners' boundaries and desires. Brainstorm creative solutions that allow each partner to feel heard and respected.

4. Respecting Autonomy:

Respecting each other's autonomy is essential for maintaining a healthy and balanced relationship. Here are some strategies to promote individual freedom and autonomy:

a. Encourage Independence: Nurture and encourage independence in each partner. Support individual hobbies, interests, and personal goals. Recognize that maintaining a sense of self outside of the relationship is crucial for personal growth and fulfillment.

b. Mutual Support: Provide support and encouragement for each other's individual pursuits. Celebrate each other's achievements and show interest in each other's personal growth. This strengthens the bond by fostering an environment of mutual support and encouragement.

c. Balance Togetherness and Independence: Find a healthy balance between spending time together and having individual time. Respect each other's need for alone time or time spent with friends and family. Strive for a balance that allows for both togetherness and individuality.
d. Practice Trust: Trust is fundamental to honoring individual desires and boundaries. Trust that your partner's desires and boundaries are valid and important. Avoid controlling or manipulative behaviors that undermine trust and autonomy.

Honoring individual desires and boundaries is crucial for maintaining a healthy, respectful, and fulfilling relationship. By fostering open communication, setting and respecting boundaries, practicing effective communication and negotiation, and respecting each other's autonomy, couples can create an environment that nurtures individual needs and desires. Remember that honoring individual desires and boundaries is an ongoing process that requires active effort and regular check-ins. Embrace the uniqueness of each partner and celebrate the diverse desires and boundaries within your relationship. By doing so, you can create a strong and harmonious connection that allows for personal growth, satisfaction, and a deep sense of mutual respect.

4.2 Mutual Exploration and Shared Fantasies

Mutual exploration and shared fantasies are powerful ways to deepen intimacy and connection within a relationship. They provide an opportunity for couples to explore new dimensions of pleasure, enhance communication, and foster a sense of adventure and playfulness. In this chapter, we will delve into the importance of mutual exploration and shared fantasies, and provide strategies for creating a safe and exciting space to explore together.

1. Understanding Mutual Exploration:

Mutual exploration involves embarking on a journey of discovery together, where both partners actively engage in exploring new experiences, desires, and fantasies. Here are key points to consider:

a. Embracing Openness: Cultivate an environment of openness and acceptance, where both partners feel comfortable expressing their desires and curiosities. Create a safe space where you can explore without judgment or fear of rejection.

b. Curiosity and Adventure: Foster a sense of curiosity and adventure within the relationship. Encourage each other to explore new experiences, whether they are sexual or non-sexual. Embrace a mindset of lifelong learning and discovery.

c. Active Consent: Prioritize active and enthusiastic consent. Always seek consent from your partner before engaging in any new activity or exploring a shared fantasy. Regularly check in with each other to ensure ongoing consent and comfort.

d. Mutual Satisfaction: Mutual exploration should be focused on the satisfaction and pleasure of both partners. Strive for a balanced approach where both partners' desires and boundaries are respected and fulfilled.

2. Creating a Safe Space:

Creating a safe space for mutual exploration is essential for partners to feel comfortable expressing their desires and fantasies. Here are strategies to establish a safe and trusting environment:

a. Open and Non-judgmental Communication: Foster open and non-judgmental communication about desires, fantasies, and boundaries. Encourage active listening, empathy, and understanding. Create a judgment-free zone where both partners feel heard and respected.
b. Establishing Boundaries: Clearly communicate and respect each other's boundaries. Discuss and agree upon limits and boundaries before engaging in any new exploration. Regularly check in with each other to ensure that boundaries are being honored.
c. Safe Words or Signals: Establish safe words or signals that can be used to pause or stop any activity during exploration. These provide a clear and effective way for either partner to communicate their comfort levels and ensure that boundaries are respected.
d. Building Trust: Mutual exploration requires a foundation of trust. Invest time and effort in building trust within the relationship. Trust allows for vulnerability, openness, and a sense of safety in exploring shared fantasies and desires.

3. Sharing Fantasies:

Shared fantasies can be a powerful tool for deepening intimacy and connection. They provide an opportunity to explore desires and create a unique bond between partners. Here are strategies for sharing fantasies:

a. Create a Judgment-Free Zone: Foster an environment where both partners feel safe sharing their fantasies without fear of judgment or criticism. Embrace an attitude of acceptance and curiosity, valuing each other's desires.

b. Open and Honest Conversations: Engage in open and honest conversations about fantasies. Encourage each other to share desires, exploring the emotional and psychological aspects behind them. Practice active listening and validate each other's fantasies.

c. Respect Boundaries and Consent: Ensure that shared fantasies align with both partners' boundaries and comfort levels. Consent should always be obtained before incorporating any fantasy into the relationship. Regularly check in with each other to ensure ongoing consent and mutual satisfaction.

d. Explore Creative Outlets: Find creative outlets to explore shared fantasies. This could include role-playing, erotic storytelling, watching or reading erotic material together, or creating a shared fantasy board where you can both contribute ideas.

4. Experimenting with New Experiences:

Mutual exploration often involves experimenting with new experiences to fulfill shared fantasies and desires. Here are strategies for introducing and navigating new experiences:

a. Start Slowly: Begin with small steps and gradually increase the intensity or complexity of new experiences. This allows both partners to adjust and communicate their comfort levels effectively.

b. Mutual Agreement: Ensure that both partners are equally enthusiastic about trying new experiences. Avoid pressuring or coercing your partner into activities they are not comfortable with.

c. Regular Check-Ins: Regularly check in with each other during and after new experiences. Discuss how it felt, what worked, and what didn't. This ongoing feedback ensures that both partners feel heard and respected.

d. Learning and Growing Together: View new experiences as opportunities for growth and learning. Embrace any challenges as opportunities for deeper connection and understanding within the relationship.

Mutual exploration and shared fantasies can greatly enhance intimacy, connection, and pleasure within a relationship. By creating a safe space, engaging in open communication, and respecting each other's boundaries and desires, couples can embark on a journey of mutual discovery and fulfillment. Remember that mutual exploration is a collaborative process that requires ongoing consent, communication, and respect for individual comfort levels. Embrace the excitement of exploring new experiences together and enjoy the deepening intimacy that comes from sharing fantasies and desires.

4.3 Intimacy Beyond the Bedroom

While the bedroom often serves as the primary space for physical intimacy in a relationship, true connection and intimacy can extend far beyond the confines of that space. Intimacy encompasses emotional, intellectual, and spiritual connection, and it is important to nurture these aspects of your relationship outside of the bedroom as well. In this chapter, we will explore the various ways to cultivate intimacy beyond the bedroom, fostering a deeper bond and enhancing the overall connection between partners.

1. Emotional Intimacy:

Emotional intimacy forms the foundation of a strong and meaningful relationship. It involves sharing and understanding each other's emotions, vulnerabilities, and deepest desires. Here are strategies for nurturing emotional intimacy:

a. Open Communication: Foster open and honest communication about your feelings, thoughts, and experiences. Practice active listening and empathize with your partner's emotions. Create a safe space where you can express yourselves without fear of judgment or rejection.

b. Vulnerability and Trust: Allow yourselves to be vulnerable with each other. Share your fears, insecurities, and dreams. Building trust is crucial for creating an environment where emotional intimacy can flourish.

c. Quality Time: Set aside dedicated time for meaningful conversations and bonding activities. This could include date nights, shared hobbies, or simply spending quality time together without distractions. Focus on connecting deeply and genuinely with each other.

d. Express Appreciation and Gratitude: Regularly express appreciation and gratitude for each other. Acknowledge and validate each other's efforts, qualities, and contributions to the relationship. This fosters a sense of emotional connection and appreciation.

2. Intellectual Intimacy:

Intellectual intimacy involves engaging in stimulating conversations, sharing ideas, and cultivating a sense of intellectual connection. Here are strategies for nurturing intellectual intimacy:

a. Engage in Intellectual Discussions: Discuss various topics of interest, such as current events, books, movies, or shared hobbies. Encourage each other's intellectual growth and curiosity. Explore new ideas and perspectives together.
b. Collaborative Projects: Engage in collaborative projects or activities that allow you to work together towards a common goal. This could include planning a trip, starting a creative project, or solving puzzles. Collaboration fosters intellectual connection and strengthens teamwork.
c. Learn Together: Pursue opportunities for learning and personal growth as a couple. Take classes, attend workshops or seminars, or explore new areas of knowledge together. This shared learning experience deepens intellectual intimacy.
d. Share Personal Insights: Share your personal insights, thoughts, and reflections with each other. Engage in deep conversations that challenge and inspire both partners. Embrace the opportunity to learn from each other's unique perspectives.

3. Spiritual Intimacy:

Spiritual intimacy involves connecting on a deeper level of shared values, beliefs, and purpose. It is about nurturing a sense of spirituality or shared meaning within the relationship. Here are strategies for nurturing spiritual intimacy:

a. Explore Shared Values: Engage in conversations about your shared values and beliefs. Discuss what gives your life meaning and purpose. Identify and celebrate the shared spiritual elements in your relationship.
b. Practice Mindfulness and Presence: Cultivate a sense of mindfulness and presence in your interactions. Practice activities such as meditation, yoga, or nature walk together. These activities can deepen your connection and create space for spiritual exploration.
c. Rituals and Traditions: Establish rituals or traditions that hold spiritual significance for both partners. This could include practicing gratitude together, creating a shared spiritual space in your home, or participating in rituals that resonate with your beliefs.
d. Support Each Other's Spiritual Growth: Encourage and support each other's spiritual growth and exploration. Respect and honor each other's individual spiritual paths, even if they differ. Seek opportunities to learn from and inspire each other spiritually.

4. Physical Affection and Non-sexual Intimacy:

Physical affection plays a vital role in nurturing intimacy beyond the bedroom. It involves expressing love, care, and connection through touch and non-sexual intimacy. Here are strategies for fostering physical affection and non-sexual intimacy:

a. Hugs, Kisses, and Cuddles: Incorporate regular hugs, kisses, and cuddling into your daily routines. These acts of physical affection can convey love, warmth, and security.

b. Non-sexual Touch: Engage in non-sexual touches, such as holding hands, giving massages, or stroking each other's hair. Physical touch can deepen the emotional connection and create a sense of closeness.

c. Engage in Shared Activities: Participate in activities that promote physical connection, such as dancing, exercising together, or taking walks hand in hand. These shared experiences strengthen the bond between partners.

d. Show Appreciation through Touch: Use touch to show appreciation and affection. A gentle touch on the arm or a loving pat on the back can convey love and support.

Intimacy beyond the bedroom is essential for fostering a deep and meaningful connection in a relationship. By nurturing emotional intimacy, engaging in intellectual discussions, exploring spirituality together, and fostering physical affection and non-sexual intimacy, couples can strengthen their bond and create a sense of closeness that extends far beyond the confines of the bedroom. Remember that each aspect of intimacy requires ongoing effort, communication, and mutual understanding. Embrace the opportunity to explore and cultivate intimacy in various areas of your relationship, and enjoy the profound connection that comes from sharing your lives holistically.

4.4 Rekindling Passion and Spark in Long-Term Relationships

Long-term relationships are a beautiful journey of growth, love, and companionship. However, over time, the initial spark and passion can fade, leaving couples yearning to reignite the flame. Rekindling passion and spark in a long-term relationship requires effort, creativity, and a willingness to explore new avenues of connection. In this chapter, we will explore strategies for reigniting passion and infusing excitement into a long-term relationship.

1. Prioritizing Quality Time:

Quality time is essential for nurturing passion and intimacy in a long-term relationship. Here are strategies to prioritize quality time together:

a. Date Nights: Set aside dedicated date nights to spend quality time together. Plan activities that you both enjoy and that promote connection and enjoyment. This can range from going out for a romantic dinner to engaging in fun and adventurous activities.

b. Unplug and Connect: Disconnect from technology and distractions to fully engage with each other. Create sacred spaces where you can focus solely on each other and deepen your connection.

c. Shared Interests: Discover new shared interests or revisit old ones. Engage in activities that bring you joy and allow you to bond on a deeper level. This could include hobbies, sports, or creative endeavors.

d. Emotional Check-Ins: Regularly check in with each other on an emotional level. Ask meaningful questions and actively listen to your partner's responses. Show genuine interest in their thoughts, feelings, and experiences.

2. Communication and Emotional Intimacy:

Effective communication and emotional intimacy are essential for reigniting passion in a long-term relationship. Here are strategies for fostering open and intimate communication:

a. Express Desires and Fantasies: Share your desires and fantasies with each other in a safe and non-judgmental environment. Explore the possibility of incorporating these desires into your intimate experiences.
b. Active Listening: Practice active listening by giving your partner your full attention and responding with empathy. Create a space where both partners feel heard and understood.
c. Share Appreciation and Affection: Express appreciation and affection for each other regularly. Vocalize your love, admiration, and gratitude for your partner's qualities and actions.
d. Emotional Vulnerability: Create a safe space for emotional vulnerability. Encourage each other to share fears, dreams, and concerns. Embrace vulnerability as an opportunity for a deeper connection.

3. Spontaneity and Novelty:

Introducing spontaneity and novelty can inject excitement and passion back into a long-term relationship. Here are strategies to infuse spontaneity into your relationship:

a. Surprise Gestures: Surprise your partner with small gestures of love and thoughtfulness. This could include leaving a love note, planning a surprise outing, or preparing their favorite meal.
b. Explore New Experiences: Break free from routine and try new experiences together. This could involve traveling to new destinations, trying new activities, or exploring different cuisines.
c. Role-playing and Fantasy: Engage in role-playing or explore shared fantasies to introduce a sense of novelty and excitement into the bedroom. Ensure both partners are comfortable and consenting.
d. Adventure and Playfulness: Embrace a spirit of adventure and playfulness in your relationship. Engage in playful activities, engage in friendly competition, or embark on adventures together.

4. Physical Intimacy and Sensuality:

Physical intimacy and sensuality are vital components of passion in a long-term relationship. Here are strategies for reigniting physical intimacy:

a. Prioritize Intimate Moments: Set aside dedicated time for physical intimacy. Create a sensual environment that allows you to connect on a deep and intimate level.
b. Sensate Focus: Engage in sensate focus exercises, where the focus is on the physical sensations of touch and pleasure. Slow down and

explore each other's bodies without the pressure of sexual performance.

c. Sensual Exploration: Experiment with new techniques, positions, or intimate activities that bring pleasure and excitement to both partners. Communication and consent are key in exploring new boundaries.

d. Emotional Connection during Intimacy: Cultivate emotional connection during intimate moments by maintaining eye contact, expressing love and appreciation, and focusing on each other's pleasure and satisfaction.

Rekindling passion and spark in a long-term relationship requires dedication, effort, and a willingness to explore new avenues of connection. By prioritizing quality time, fostering open communication and emotional intimacy, introducing spontaneity and novelty, and nurturing physical intimacy and sensuality, couples can reignite the flame and infuse excitement into their relationship. Remember that each relationship is unique, and it's essential to find strategies that resonate with both partners. Embrace the journey of rediscovery, and enjoy the profound connection and passion that can be rekindled in a long-term relationship.

Chapter 5: Transforming Relationships

Relationships are dynamic entities that go through various phases and stages of growth. Transforming a relationship involves consciously working towards positive changes, growth, and evolution. In this chapter, we will explore strategies for transforming relationships, fostering deeper connections, and creating a fulfilling partnership.

1. Self-Reflection and Personal Growth:

Transformation in a relationship begins with self-reflection and personal growth. Here are strategies to foster personal growth within the context of a relationship:

a. Self-Awareness: Cultivate self-awareness by exploring your own strengths, weaknesses, values, and beliefs. Understand your patterns, triggers, and areas for personal development.

b. Self-Care: Prioritize self-care and well-being. Take care of your physical, mental, and emotional health, as it positively impacts your overall relationship dynamics.

c. Continuous Learning: Embrace a mindset of continuous learning and personal growth. Engage in activities that promote self-improvement, such as reading, attending workshops, or seeking therapy or counseling.

d. Personal Goals: Set and pursue personal goals that align with your values and aspirations. Having a sense of individual purpose and fulfillment enhances the overall quality of the relationship.

2. Cultivating Empathy and Compassion:

Empathy and compassion are vital for transforming relationships. Here are strategies to cultivate empathy and compassion within the relationship:

a. Active Listening: Practice active listening, seeking to understand your partner's perspectives, feelings, and needs. Avoid judgment or defensiveness, and validate their experiences.
b. Perspective-Taking: Put yourself in your partner's shoes and try to understand their point of view. Empathize with their emotions and experiences, even if you may not fully agree.
c. Practice Kindness: Engage in acts of kindness towards your partner. Small gestures of love, care, and appreciation can go a long way in fostering compassion and connection.
d. Emotional Support: Provide emotional support to your partner during challenging times. Show empathy, offer a safe space for them to express themselves, and validate their emotions.

3. Conflict Resolution and Communication:

Transforming a relationship involves improving conflict resolution skills and communication patterns. Here are strategies to enhance conflict resolution and communication:

a. Constructive Communication: Foster open and constructive communication by using "I" statements, expressing feelings and needs, and avoiding blame or criticism. Focus on finding solutions together.

b. Active Conflict Resolution: Develop healthy conflict resolution skills, such as active listening, compromise, and finding win-win solutions. Seek to understand the underlying causes of conflict and work towards resolution.

c. Healthy Boundaries: Establish and respect healthy boundaries within the relationship. Clearly communicate your needs, expectations, and limits. Encourage your partner to do the same.

d. Seek Professional Help: If communication or conflict resolution becomes challenging, consider seeking the guidance of a therapist or counselor who specializes in relationships. Professional support can provide valuable tools and insights.

4. Shared Goals and Mutual Growth:

Transformation in a relationship involves setting shared goals and supporting each other's growth. Here are strategies for shared goals and mutual growth:

a. Relationship Vision: Create a shared vision for the relationship. Discuss and align your long-term goals, values, and aspirations. Work together towards a common purpose.

b. Supportive Environment: Foster an environment that supports each other's individual growth and goals. Celebrate each other's achievements and provide encouragement and support.

c. Collaborative Decision-Making: Involve each other in decision-making processes that impact the relationship. Embrace compromise, respect different perspectives, and find mutually beneficial solutions.

d. Continued Exploration and Adventure: Maintain a sense of curiosity and adventure within the relationship. Explore new experiences, travel together, and seek opportunities for shared growth and discovery.

Transforming a relationship requires commitment, self-reflection, and a willingness to evolve and grow. By fostering personal growth, cultivating empathy and compassion, improving conflict resolution and communication skills, and setting shared goals for mutual growth, couples can create a fulfilling and transformative partnership. Remember that transformation is an ongoing process that requires consistent effort, patience, and understanding. Embrace the journey of transformation, and enjoy the profound connection and growth that can be achieved within your relationship.

5.2 Embracing the Power of Seduction

Seduction is an art that has been celebrated throughout history for its ability to ignite desire, passion, and connection between individuals. Embracing the power of seduction can add excitement, intimacy, and a sense of playfulness to a relationship. In this chapter, we will explore strategies for harnessing the power of seduction to enhance the bond between partners and create a captivating and enticing dynamic.

1. Understanding Seduction:

Before diving into the strategies, it's important to understand the essence of seduction. Seduction is not merely about physical attraction or manipulation. It is about creating an irresistible allure that draws someone in emotionally, mentally, and physically. Seduction is a dance of anticipation, exploration, and mutual consent.

  a. Connection and Chemistry: Seduction thrives on connection and chemistry between partners. It involves building a strong foundation of trust, emotional intimacy, and mutual understanding.
  b. Mindful Presence: Being present at the moment is essential for effective seduction. Pay attention to your partner's cues, desires, and boundaries. Be fully engaged and attuned to their needs.
  c. Confidence and Authenticity: Seduction stems from self-confidence and authenticity. Embrace and showcase your unique qualities, expressing yourself with sincerity and genuine interest in your partner.
  d. Mutual Consent: Consent is paramount in seduction. Always seek and respect your partner's boundaries and ensure that both parties are comfortable and enthusiastically engaged in the seductive experience.

2. Cultivating Sensuality:

Sensuality is at the heart of seduction. It involves engaging all the senses to create a captivating and pleasurable experience. Here are strategies for cultivating sensuality:

  a. Dress to Impress: Pay attention to your appearance and dress in a way that makes you feel confident and attractive. Consider your partner's preferences and dress in a way that entices their desires.
  b. Enhancing the Environment: Create a sensual atmosphere by setting the mood with lighting, music, and scents. Use soft lighting,

play sensual music, and incorporate enticing aromas to awaken the senses.

c. Mindful Touch: Explore the power of touch to ignite desire. Use gentle caresses, soft kisses, and playful touches to create anticipation and build excitement.

d. Sensual Indulgences: Indulge in sensual experiences together, such as sharing a decadent meal, enjoying a sensuous massage, or engaging in activities that heighten pleasure and connection.

3. Flirting and Playfulness:

Flirting and playfulness are key components of seduction. They create a sense of intrigue, excitement, and lightheartedness within the relationship. Here are strategies for incorporating flirting and playfulness:

a. Playful Banter: Engage in light-hearted teasing, witty remarks, and playful banter. This creates a playful and flirtatious dynamic between partners.

b. Unexpected Surprises: Surprise your partner with unexpected gestures that evoke excitement and anticipation. This could include leaving flirtatious notes, planning surprise outings, or initiating spontaneous activities.

c. Eye Contact and Body Language: Use eye contact and body language to convey your interest and desire. Maintain eye contact during conversations and use subtle gestures and postures to communicate attraction.

d. Humor and Laughter: Embrace humor and laughter as powerful tools of seduction. Share jokes, funny stories, and humorous moments to create a joyful and relaxed atmosphere.

4. Communication and Fantasy:

Effective communication and the exploration of fantasies can heighten the seductive experience. Here are strategies for incorporating communication and fantasy into seduction:

a. Open Communication: Share your desires, fantasies, and preferences with your partner. Create a safe space where both partners can openly express their wants and needs.
b. Role-Playing and Fantasy Exploration: Explore role-playing scenarios and fantasies together, where both partners can take on different personas and engage in playful exploration.
c. Erotic Communication: Engage in seductive and flirtatious communication, such as exchanging provocative messages, engaging in sensual phone calls, or writing passionate love letters.
d. Active Listening: Pay attention to your partner's desires and fantasies. Actively listen and respond to their needs, creating a collaborative and fulfilling seductive experience.

Embracing the power of seduction can bring a sense of thrill, passion, and connection to a relationship. By understanding the essence of seduction, cultivating sensuality, incorporating flirting and playfulness, and embracing communication and fantasy, couples can enhance their intimate experiences and create a captivating and enticing dynamic. Remember that seduction is a consensual and mutually enjoyable experience, where both partners actively participate in creating desire and passion. Explore, experiment, and embrace the art of seduction as a powerful tool for deepening intimacy and strengthening the bond between you and your partner.

5.2 Elevating Foreplay and Sexual Tension

Foreplay is a crucial component of a satisfying and fulfilling sexual experience. It builds anticipation, heightens arousal, and deepens the connection between partners. Elevating foreplay and sexual tension can take intimate moments to new levels of pleasure and intensity. In this chapter, we will explore strategies for enhancing foreplay and creating an atmosphere of sexual tension that intensifies the overall sexual experience.

1. Understanding the Importance of Foreplay:

Foreplay is not just a prelude to intercourse; it is an integral part of the sexual experience. It prepares the mind and body for pleasure, enhances arousal, and fosters intimacy. Here are some reasons why foreplay is important:

a. Arousal and Sensitization: Foreplay helps to awaken the body's arousal mechanisms and increase sensitivity to touch, making the subsequent sexual experience more pleasurable.
b. Emotional Connection: Engaging in foreplay allows partners to connect emotionally and deepen their bond. It fosters intimacy, trust, and a sense of mutual exploration.
c. Exploration and Communication: Foreplay provides an opportunity to explore each other's desires, preferences, and boundaries. It allows for open communication and the discovery of new sensations and pleasures.
d. Orgasmic Potential: Building sexual tension through foreplay can lead to more intense and satisfying orgasms for both partners.

2. Building Anticipation and Sexual Tension:

Sexual tension is the build-up of desire and anticipation between partners. It creates a heightened sense of excitement and longing, making the eventual release more intense. Here are strategies for building anticipation and sexual tension:

a. Flirting and Teasing: Engage in playful flirting and teasing throughout the day, even when you're not physically together. Send seductive messages or leave hints of what's to come, creating a sense of anticipation.
b. Delayed Gratification: Slow down the pace and intentionally delay the progression towards intercourse. Focus on pleasurable activities like kissing, caressing, and oral stimulation, drawing out the experience and building anticipation.
c. Sensual Descriptions: Use descriptive language to talk about desires, fantasies, and what you plan to do to each other. Verbalize your intentions in a seductive and tantalizing manner, heightening anticipation and sexual tension.
d. Provocative Touch: Incorporate light and teasing touches that evoke desire without fully satisfying it. Explore erogenous zones, lightly graze sensitive areas, or use feather-like touches to create a heightened sense of anticipation.

3. Exploring Erotic Massage:

Erotic massage can be a powerful tool for enhancing foreplay and increasing sexual tension. It combines the power of touch, relaxation, and sensuality. Here are strategies for exploring erotic massage:

a. Set the Mood: Create a comfortable and sensual environment by dimming the lights, using scented candles, and playing soft, relaxing music. Prepare warm massage oil or lotion for a smooth and pleasurable experience.
b. Slow and Deliberate Touch: Begin the massage with slow and deliberate strokes, using varying pressure and techniques. Explore different areas of the body, paying attention to erogenous zones and sensitive areas.
c. Incorporate Teasing: Introduce teasing touches and caresses that increase arousal and build sexual tension. Lightly brush against erogenous zones or use intermittent pauses to create anticipation.
d. Communication and Feedback: Maintain open communication throughout the massage. Ask for feedback from your partner and adjust your techniques accordingly. Encourage your partner to express their desires and preferences.

4. Incorporating Sensory Play:

Sensory play involves stimulating the senses to enhance pleasure and intensify the sexual experience. It can add excitement, anticipation, and a new level of sensuality to foreplay. Here are strategies for incorporating sensory play:

a. Blindfolding: Use a blindfold to temporarily deprive your partner of sight, intensifying their other senses. This heightens anticipation and increases sensitivity to touch, sound, and smell.
b. Temperature Play: Experiment with hot and cold sensations by using ice cubes, warm oils, or heated massage stones. Alternate between different temperatures to create contrast and heighten arousal.

c. Aromatherapy: Use scented oils, candles, or incense with aphrodisiac properties to create a sensual ambiance. Explore fragrances such as jasmine, ylang-ylang, or sandalwood known for their arousing qualities.

d. Erotic Food Play: Incorporate edible items into foreplay, such as whipped cream, chocolate sauce, or fruits. Use them to tease and tantalize your partner's body, creating a playful and sensual experience.

Elevating foreplay and sexual tension can significantly enhance the overall sexual experience and deepen the connection between partners. By understanding the importance of foreplay, building anticipation and sexual tension, exploring erotic massage, and incorporating sensory play, couples can create a heightened sense of pleasure, intimacy, and satisfaction. Remember to communicate openly, prioritize consent, and continuously explore and adapt these techniques to suit your unique desires and boundaries. Embrace the journey of deepening intimacy through elevated foreplay and enjoy the intensified pleasure and connection it brings to your relationship.

5.3 Exploring Sexual Positions and Variations

Sexual positions and variations play a vital role in the exploration and enjoyment of sexual intimacy. They allow couples to discover new sensations, increase pleasure, and enhance their physical connection. In this chapter, we will explore a range of sexual positions and variations that can add excitement, novelty, and pleasure to your intimate encounters.

1. Importance of Sexual Positions:

Sexual positions not only offer physical variety but also allow for deeper penetration, clitoral stimulation, and access to erogenous zones. They can enhance intimacy, facilitate communication, and provide opportunities for both partners to experience pleasure. Here's why sexual positions are important:

a. Variety and Novelty: Exploring different positions adds variety and novelty to your sexual experiences. It keeps the excitement alive and prevents monotony in the bedroom.
b. Enhanced Stimulation: Different positions provide varying levels of clitoral, G-spot, and penile stimulation. Experimenting with positions can help you find the ones that work best for you and your partner.
c. Visual Appeal: Certain positions offer visual stimulation, allowing partners to witness each other's pleasure and intensify the erotic experience.
d. Emotional Connection: Trying new positions can foster communication, trust, and intimacy. It allows couples to openly express their desires, boundaries, and preferences.

2. Classic Sexual Positions:

a. Missionary: This position involves the partner on top, facing each other. It allows for deep penetration, eye contact, and intimate connection.

b. Doggy Style: In this position, the receiving partner is on all fours while the penetrating partner enters from behind. It offers deep penetration and allows for G-spot stimulation.

c. Cowgirl: The receiving partner straddles the penetrating partner, facing them. This position provides the receiving partner with control over the depth and pace of penetration.

d. Spooning: Partners lie on their sides, with the penetrating partner entering from behind. It offers intimate contact, and closeness, and is particularly comfortable for longer sessions.

3. Exploring New Positions and Variations:

a. Standing Positions: Try positions that involve standing, such as the Standing Doggy Style or the Wall-Supported Standing Position. These positions provide a different angle of penetration and can be exhilarating.

b. Oral Pleasure Positions: Experiment with various positions for oral sex, such as the 69 positions or the Elevated Oral Position. These positions allow for mutual pleasure and exploration.

c. Acrobatic Positions: For the more adventurous couples, acrobatic positions like the Lotus, the Wheelbarrow, or the Spider can provide a thrilling and intense experience. These positions require strength, flexibility, and trust.

d. Furniture and Prop-Assisted Positions: Incorporate furniture or props to enhance your positions. For example, using a chair for support or adding cushions to change the angle of penetration can add excitement and comfort.

4. Intimacy and Eye Contact:

a. Face-to-Face Positions: Explore positions that allow for prolonged eye contacts, such as the Deep Glider or the Yab-Yum. These positions enhance emotional connection and intimacy during sex.
b. Mirror Play: Place a mirror strategically to allow you and your partner to watch yourselves during sex. It adds visual stimulation, intensifies the experience, and creates a sense of eroticism.
c. Tantra-inspired Positions: Incorporate Tantra-inspired positions, such as the Union of the Bee, the Lotus Blossom, or the Wheel of Love. These positions focus on deep connection, energy exchange, and extended pleasure.

5. Communication and Experimentation:

a. Open Communication: Talk openly with your partner about your desires, fantasies, and preferences when it comes to sexual positions. Discuss any concerns or limitations, ensuring both partners are comfortable and consenting.
b. Experimentation: Don't be afraid to try new positions and variations. Explore different angles, depths, and speeds to find what feels best for you and your partner. Remember, it's about pleasure and enjoyment, so be open to adapting and refining as you go.

Exploring sexual positions and variations can add excitement, pleasure, and novelty to your intimate experiences. Whether you're trying classic positions, experimenting with new ones, incorporating props or furniture, or focusing on intimacy and eye contact, the key is open communication, trust, and a willingness to explore together. Remember that sexual positions should prioritize the comfort, pleasure, and consent of both partners. Embrace the joy of discovery, communicate your desires, and enjoy the journey of exploring the vast array of sexual positions and variations available to you.

5.4 Cultivating Lasting Desire and Love

Maintaining lasting desire and love in a relationship is a journey that requires effort, understanding, and continuous nurturing. While the initial spark of passion may fade over time, it is possible to cultivate a deep and enduring connection that keeps desire alive. In this chapter, we will explore strategies for cultivating lasting desire and love, fostering a fulfilling and passionate relationship.

1. **Embracing Emotional Intimacy:**

   a. Open Communication: Communication is the foundation of a strong relationship. Foster open and honest communication by actively listening to your partner, expressing your needs and desires, and creating a safe space for open dialogue.
   b. Emotional Vulnerability: Share your feelings, fears, and dreams with your partner. Allow yourself to be vulnerable, fostering a deeper emotional connection and understanding.
   c. Quality Time: Spend quality time together, free from distractions. Engage in activities that promote emotional bonding, such as taking walks, sharing meals, or engaging in shared hobbies.

d. Emotional Support: Show empathy and support for your partner's emotional well-being. Be there for them during both the highs and lows, offering a safe and nurturing space to lean on.

2. Prioritizing Physical Intimacy:

a. Intimate Touch: Engage in non-sexual physical touch regularly, such as cuddling, holding hands, or hugging. Physical touch fosters a sense of closeness, connection, and intimacy.
b. Intimacy Rituals: Create rituals that focus on physical intimacy, such as having regular date nights, setting aside time for sensual massages, or exploring new forms of physical pleasure together.
c. Spontaneity and Surprise: Inject spontaneity and surprise into your physical intimacy. Surprise your partner with affectionate gestures, love notes, or spontaneous acts of passion to keep the spark alive.
d. Sexual Exploration: Continuously explore and experiment with your sexual desires and fantasies as a couple. Be open to trying new experiences, positions, or activities that bring pleasure and excitement into the bedroom.

3. Nurturing Emotional and Physical Connection:

a. Shared Goals and Dreams: Create shared goals and dreams as a couple. Work together towards a common vision, fostering a sense of partnership and shared purpose.
b. Gratitude and Appreciation: Express gratitude and appreciation for your partner regularly. Acknowledge their efforts, strengths, and contributions, nurturing a positive and loving atmosphere.

c. Surprise Gestures of Love: Surprise your partner with gestures that show your love and appreciation. It can be as simple as leaving a love note, planning a surprise date, or cooking their favorite meal.

d. Intimate Communication: Foster intimate communication by expressing love, desire, and admiration for your partner. Verbalize your affection and appreciation, creating a nurturing and loving environment.

4. Sustaining Passion and Desire:

a. Novelty and Adventure: Inject novelty and adventure into your relationship. Explore new activities, travel together, or try new hobbies as a couple. Novel experiences can reignite passion and desire.

b. Fantasy and Imagination: Encourage each other to share fantasies and desires. Incorporate fantasy role-playing or create a shared fantasy world that allows for imaginative and passionate exploration.

c. Surprise Dates and Experiences: Plan surprise dates or experiences that keep the element of surprise and excitement alive. Explore new places, try new cuisines, or indulge in adventurous activities together.

d. Continuous Self-Growth: Focus on personal growth and self-care, both individually and as a couple. When you invest in your own well-being, you bring more fulfillment and vitality to the relationship.

5. Commitment and Effort:

a. Emotional Investment: Make a conscious commitment to the relationship and invest emotionally in its growth and well-being. Show up consistently, even during challenging times.
b. Mutual Support: Be each other's biggest supporters. Encourage and motivate each other to pursue individual goals and aspirations, fostering a sense of admiration and mutual growth.
c. Relationship Rituals: Create rituals that strengthen your bond, such as weekly check-ins, regular date nights, or annual relationship reviews. These rituals provide space for reflection, growth, and celebration.
d. Adaptability and Flexibility: Embrace change and be flexible in adapting to the evolving needs and desires of your partner and the relationship itself. This willingness to adapt fosters a sense of security and stability.

Cultivating lasting desire and love requires consistent effort, dedication, and a willingness to explore and grow together. By embracing emotional intimacy, prioritizing physical intimacy, nurturing emotional and physical connection, sustaining passion and desire, and committing to the relationship, you can create a deep and fulfilling bond that stands the test of time. Remember, cultivating lasting desire and love is an ongoing journey, and with patience, understanding, and continuous nurturing, you can create a passionate and loving relationship that grows stronger with each passing day.

Conclusion:

In conclusion, "Kama Sutra: The Modern Guide to Exploring Sensual Secrets for Transforming Relationships and Exploring the Depths of the Kama Sutra" offers a comprehensive and contemporary perspective on the ancient text, providing valuable insights and practical guidance for individuals and couples seeking to enhance their relationships and embrace a more fulfilling and sensual connection.

Throughout this book, we have delved into the historical background and origins of the Kama Sutra, understanding its key principles, and exploring its relevance in modern relationships. We have discussed building strong foundations through emotional connection, trust, and communication, as well as nurturing intimacy, vulnerability, and compatibility.

The chapters on sensual exploration have expanded the definition of sensuality, awakening the senses, and exploring pleasure techniques and erotic arts. We have also explored the incorporation of Tantra into modern relationships, enriching the spiritual and sexual connection between partners.

Deepening intimacy and connection has been a focal point, emphasizing the importance of honoring individual desires and boundaries, mutual exploration, and shared fantasies. Additionally, we have explored intimacy beyond the bedroom, rekindling passion in long-term relationships, and transforming relationships through the power of seduction.

The final chapters have delved into elevating foreplay and sexual tension, cultivating lasting desire and love, and exploring sexual positions and variations. These topics have provided practical tools, insights, and inspiration for couples to navigate the intricate dynamics of physical and emotional intimacy.

By embracing the teachings and principles of the Kama Sutra, couples can embark on a transformative journey of self-discovery, self-expression, and sensual exploration. It is a testament to the enduring relevance of this ancient text that its wisdom continues to resonate in modern relationships, guiding us toward deeper connections, heightened pleasure, and lasting love.

As we conclude this book, it is important to remember that the Kama Sutra is not a rigid set of rules, but rather a guide for individuals and couples to adapt and explore within the context of their own unique relationships. It is through open-mindedness, communication, and a willingness to embrace new experiences that we can truly unlock the transformative power of the Kama Sutra.

May this book serve as a catalyst for personal growth, deepening connection, and the exploration of sensuality and pleasure within the context of loving relationships. Let us embark on this journey together, embracing the sensual secrets and wisdom of the Kama Sutra, and transforming our relationships into vibrant, fulfilling, and transformative experiences of love, passion, and connection.